Minimally Invasive Spine Surgery Techniques

Gabriel Tender
Editor

Minimally Invasive Spine Surgery Techniques

Springer

Editor
Gabriel Tender
Louisiana State University
New Orleans, LA
USA

ISBN 978-3-030-10132-9 ISBN 978-3-319-71943-6 (eBook)
https://doi.org/10.1007/978-3-319-71943-6

Softcover re-print of the Hardcover 1st edition 2018

Printed on acid-free paper

This Springer imprint is published by Springer Nature
The registered company is Springer International Publishing AG
The registered company address is: Gewerbestrasse 11, 6330 Cham, Switzerland

Contents

Contributors

Yasser Badr Badr Brain and Spine, Los Angeles, CA, USA

Niki Calina Department of Neurosurgery, "Bagdasar-Arseni" Hospital, Bucharest, Romania

Yi-Ren Chen Department of Neurosurgery, Stanford University, Stanford, CA, USA

Ian Connolly Department of Neurosurgery, Stanford University, Stanford, CA, USA

Adriana Constantinescu Universitatea de Medicina si Farmacie, Craiova, Romania

Clifford Crutcher Department of Neurosurgery, Louisiana State University Health Sciences Center, New Orleans, LA, USA

Atman Desai Department of Neurosurgery, Stanford University, Stanford, CA, USA

Anthony Digiorgio Department of Neurosurgery, Louisiana State University Health Sciences Center, New Orleans, LA, USA

Malcolm Daniel Eggart MUSC Health Neurosciences at Tidelands Health, SC, USA

Parastou Fatemi Department of Neurosurgery, Stanford University, Stanford, CA, USA

Richard G. Fessler Department of Neurosurgery, Rush University Medical Center, Chicago, IL, USA

Mihaela Florea Department of Neurosurgery, "Bagdasar-Arseni" Hospital, Bucharest, Romania

John Gachiani Mercy Neurosurgery, Des Moines, IA, USA

Silvia Gesheva Department of Neurosurgery, Louisiana State University Health Sciences Center, New Orleans, LA, USA

George M. Ghobrial Department of Neurological Surgery and The Miami Project to Cure Paralysis, Lois Pope LIFE Center, University of Miami MILLER School of Medicine, Miami, FL, USA

Saqib Hasan Department of Orthopedic Surgery, NYU Langone Health, New York, NY, USA

Mena G. Kerolus Department of Neurosurgery, Rush University Medical Center, Chicago, IL, USA

Lindsay Lasseigne Department of Neurosurgery, Louisiana State University Health Sciences Center, New Orleans, LA, USA

Allan D. Levi Department of Neurological Surgery and The Miami Project to Cure Paralysis, Lois Pope LIFE Center, University of Miami MILLER School of Medicine, Miami, FL, USA

Zachary A. Medress Department of Neurosurgery, Stanford University, Stanford, CA, USA

Joseph E. Molenda Department of Neurosurgery, Rush University Medical Center, Chicago, IL, USA

Ronald Moskovich Department of Orthopedic Surgery, NYU Langone Health, New York, NY, USA

Remi Nader Texas Center for Neurosciences PLLC, Houston, TX, USA

American Board of Neurological Surgery, Chicago, IL, USA

Division of Neurosurgery, University of Texas Medical Branch, Galveston, TX, USA

William Carey University, Hattiesburg, MS, USA

Department of Neurosurgery, Tulane University, New Orleans, LA, USA

Kara Parikh Department of Neurosurgery, Louisiana State University Health Sciences Center, New Orleans, LA, USA

John Ratliff Department of Neurosurgery, Stanford University, Stanford, CA, USA

Daniel Serban Department of Neurosurgery, "Bagdasar-Arseni" Hospital, Bucharest, Romania

Durga R. Sure Essentia Health, Duluth, MN, USA

Gabriel Tender Louisiana State University, New Orleans, LA, USA

Mazda K. Turel Department of Neurosurgery, Rush University Medical Center, Chicago, IL, USA

Anand Veeravagu Department of Neurosurgery, Stanford University, Stanford, CA, USA

Rand Voorhies Southern Brain and Spine, Metairie, LA, USA

Alexis Waguespack Spinecare Medical Group, Marrero, LA, USA

Jason Wilson Department of Neurosurgery, Louisiana State University Health Sciences Center, New Orleans, LA, USA

Chapter 1
Introduction to Minimally Invasive Spine Surgery

Gabriel Tender, Daniel Serban, and Anthony DiGiorgio

Spinal pathology is widespread in the United States and, as the population ages, the prevalence is only going to increase. Greater than 90% of adults older than 65 show radiographic evidence of spinal degeneration [1] and 25% of all adults report some sort of physical limitation due to spine problems [2]. This is one of the leading causes of emergency room visits, missed work days, disability and productivity loss in the country. The average annual health care costs of an individual with low back pain are nearly three times those of one without [3]. Overall, spinal pathology costs American society over $200 billion per year [4].

This cost will continue to grow. Expenditures for patients with spine pathology have increased faster than overall healthcare expenditures [2] (which are already expanding at an alarming rate). Millions of patients are seeking relief with conservative measures each year [5] and over a third of these patients are taking some sort of opioid pain medication [3]. However, in select patients, surgical intervention has been shown to be cost-effective, decreasing analgesic use and days missed from work [5, 6].

Advances in spine surgery continue as surgeons strive for better outcomes, leading to the advent of minimally invasive surgery (MIS). Operations that had been performed via large incisions with dissection of tendon & ligamentous attachments can now be performed using tubes, expandable retractors and microscopes (Fig. 1.1).

G. Tender (✉)
Louisiana State University, New Orleans, LA, USA

D. Serban
Department of Neurosurgery, "Bagdasar-Arseni" Hospital, Bucharest, Romania

A. DiGiorgio
Department of Neurosurgery, Louisiana State University Health Sciences Center, New Orleans, LA, USA
e-mail: Adigi2@lsuhsc.edu

G. Tender (ed.), *Minimally Invasive Spine Surgery Techniques*,
https://doi.org/10.1007/978-3-319-71943-6_1

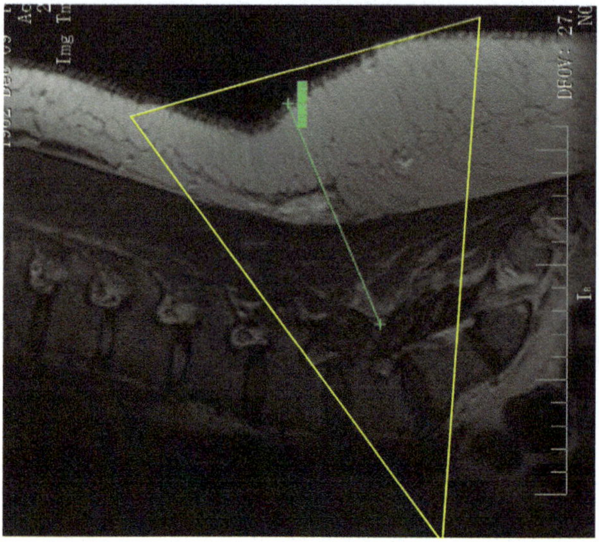

Fig. 1.1 Preoperative evaluation by lumbar MRI, suggesting the extent of the skin incision and muscle dissection necessary to access the disc in an obese patient. The same patient would be able to undergo a minimally invasive fusion through a less than 1 in. incision

These various portals minimize the disruption to the surrounding tissues, leading to less blood loss, decreased postoperative pain and faster recovery.

Advancing MIS techniques been expanded to all areas of the spine, and are not limited to degenerative disease. MIS has been utilized for neoplastic, infectious, deformity and traumatic etiologies as well. Mastery of these technologies is another tool for the surgeon's armamentarium, not meant to completely replace open surgery. In fact, algorithms have been developed to guide surgeons to the appropriate use of minimally invasive versus open surgery [7, 8].

As healthcare business models move to a more value-based paradigm, improved cost-effectiveness is needed to justify the increased upfront costs of new technologies. Additionally, MIS techniques come with a steep learning curve. The improved economic benefits of MIS are not immediately realized and there is a paucity of economic research showing a benefit of MIS [9–11]. However, as surgeons increase their experience, operative times and length of stay decrease [12]. Length of stay is one of the primary drivers in hospitalization costs after spine surgery [13], and decreasing this is sure to please patients, providers and payers alike.

While the perceived benefits of MIS are becoming more illuminated in the literature, market demands continue to push the envelope of this emerging technology. The competitive nature of modern medical practice continues to drive the delivery of surgical spine care. The ability to offer MIS techniques is becoming a requirement for today's spine surgeon.

Nonetheless, the minimally invasive spinal techniques started to blossom at the turn of the millennium and many had anticipated that they will become the standard of care within 5–10 years. We are now almost 20 years later and still the minimally invasive techniques are used and taught in academic centers in only 10–20% of all cases. So why have the surgeons not embraced and the patients not demanded the minimally invasive spine techniques?

The answers are complex and an in-depth analysis is beyond the scope of this book. However, one of the major factors playing a role in the lack of widespread usage of MIS techniques is the difficult learning curve. The minimally invasive techniques are practiced and taught by "open" surgeons who have converted to the new techniques. The problem is, even the most talented surgeons will experience a longer operative time when they first start practicing the MIS techniques. This may be frustrating and discouraging, not to mention financially detrimental for the private practice spine surgeon. Fortunately, once the surgeon becomes experienced in the MIS techniques, the operative time typically decreases below that of open cases, and we have yet to encounter a surgeon who reverted to the open techniques once the minimally invasive ones were mastered.

Probably the best time to learn the MIS techniques is in residency (like everything else in surgery, or medicine for that matter). The residents are unbiased and they will learn new things as they are introduced to them, without having to break "old habits" or worry about increased operative time and implicitly decreased revenue. We strongly believe that the residents should be exposed to both the open spinal procedures (initially) and the minimally invasive techniques, once they have a good understanding of the anatomy. It is imperative for them to learn not only the surgical skills, but also the limitations of these techniques.

This book was written for the residents and all the spine surgeons who want to better understand the minimally invasive spine surgery techniques. It was intended to offer a unique technical manual with detailed algorithms for these techniques. Each chapter provides a thorough description of the standard surgical technique, followed by pearls learned through almost 20 years of MIS experience. Finally, and probably most importantly, we selected the most representative operative videos for each chapter, in an attempt to provide a "real life" experience to the training surgeon. We hope that our readers, from the novice resident to the experienced surgeon, will find something new and interesting in this book.

References

1. Hicks GE, Morone N, Weiner DK. Degenerative lumbar disc and facet disease in older adults: prevalence and clinical correlates. Spine (Phila Pa 1976). 2009;34:1301–6.
2. Martin BI, Deyo RA, Mirza SK, Turner JA, Comstock BA, Hollingworth W, et al. Expenditures and health status among adults with back and neck problems. JAMA. 2008;299:656–64.
3. Gore M, Sadosky A, Stacey BR, Tai KS, Leslie D. The burden of chronic low back pain: clinical comorbidities, treatment patterns, and health care costs in usual care settings. Spine (Phila Pa 1976). 2012;37:E668–77.
4. Ma VY, Chan L, Carruthers KJ. Incidence, prevalence, costs, and impact on disability of common conditions requiring rehabilitation in the United States: stroke, spinal cord injury, traumatic brain injury, multiple sclerosis, osteoarthritis, rheumatoid arthritis, limb loss, and back pain. Arch Phys Med Rehabil. 2014;95:986–995.e1.

5. O'Lynnger TM, Zuckerman SL, Morone PJ, Dewan MC, Vasquez-Castellanos RA, Cheng JS. Trends for spine surgery for the elderly: implications for access to healthcare in North America. Neurosurgery. 2015;77(Suppl 4):S136–41.
6. Devin CJ, Chotai S, Parker SL, Tetreault L, Fehlings MG, McGirt MJ. A cost-utility analysis of lumbar decompression with and without fusion for degenerative spine disease in the elderly. Neurosurgery. 2015;77(Suppl 4):S116–24.
7. Dhall SS, Wadhwa R, Wang MY, Tien-Smith A, Mummaneni PV. Traumatic thoracolumbar spinal injury: an algorithm for minimally invasive surgical management. Neurosurg Focus. 2014;37:E9.
8. Mummaneni PV, Shaffrey CI, Lenke LG, Park P, Wang MY, La Marca F, et al. The minimally invasive spinal deformity surgery algorithm: a reproducible rational framework for decision making in minimally invasive spinal deformity surgery. Neurosurg Focus. 2014;36:E6.
9. Hofstetter CP, Hofer AS, Wang MY. Economic impact of minimally invasive lumbar surgery. World J Orthop. 2015;6:190–201.
10. Lubelski D, Mihalovich KE, Skelly AC, Fehlings MG, Harrop JS, Mummaneni PV, et al. Is minimal access spine surgery more cost-effective than conventional spine surgery? Spine (Phila Pa 1976). 2014;39:S65–74.
11. Parker SL, Adogwa O, Davis BJ, Fulchiero E, Aaronson O, Cheng J, et al. Cost-utility analysis of minimally invasive versus open multilevel hemilaminectomy for lumbar stenosis. J Spinal Disord Tech. 2013;26:42–7.
12. Ahn J, Iqbal A, Manning BT, Leblang S, Bohl DD, Mayo BC, et al. Minimally invasive lumbar decompression-the surgical learning curve. Spine J. 2016;16:909–16.
13. Missios S, Bekelis K. Hospitalization cost after spine surgery in the United States of America. J Clin Neurosci. 2015;22:1632–7.

Chapter 2
Microdiscectomy

Niki Calina, Daniel Serban, Adriana Constantinescu, Anthony Digiorgio, and Gabriel Tender

Introduction

Lumbar microdiscectomy performed through a tubular retractor is typically the first minimally invasive operation of spine surgeons. This technique involves an algorithm of operative steps that allows safe removal of the herniated disc with minimal complications.

Indications

The indications for lumbar minimally invasive laminotomy are the same as for the open laminotomy—unilateral lumbar stenosis with compression of a spinal nerve and resultant radiculopathy, due to one or more of the following:

- herniated nucleus pulposus
- facet or yellow ligament hypertrophy
- synovial cysts or other space occupying lesions.

Electronic Supplementary Material The online version of this chapter https://doi.org/10.1007/978-3-319-71943-6_2. contains supplementary material, which is available to authorized users.

N. Calina • D. Serban
Department of Neurosurgery, "Bagdasar-Arseni" Hospital, Bucharest, Romania

A. Constantinescu
Universitatea de Medicina si Farmacie, Craiova, Romania

A. DiGiorgio
Department of Neurosurgery, Louisiana State University Health Sciences Center, New Orleans, LA, USA
e-mail: Adigi2@lsuhsc.edu

G. Tender (✉)
Louisiana State University, New Orleans, LA, USA

G. Tender (ed.), *Minimally Invasive Spine Surgery Techniques*,
https://doi.org/10.1007/978-3-319-71943-6_2

Most surgeons recommend a short course of conservative treatment prior to surgical intervention, with the caveat that delaying the nerve decompression for more than 6 months from the onset of symptoms may result in chronic pain and/or persistent sensory/motor deficits, despite removal of the herniated disc.

Contraindications

There are no absolute contraindications for this technique.

A relative contraindication is a recurrent disc herniation that was initially treated by an open discectomy. In these cases, the same skin incision should be used. If the initial herniation was treated in a minimally invasive fashion, it should also be re-explored through the same incision, with a tubular retractor.

Another relative contraindication is morbid obesity, when the distance between the skin surface and the lamina is over 100 mm (the longest typical tubular retractor). However, since the fat is depressible, we have used this technique in many morbidly obese patients without having to convert to an open procedure.

Surgical Technique

The following operative steps are described:

- positioning
- skin incision
- retractor placement
- laminotomy
- yellow ligament removal
- discectomy
- closure

Positioning

The patient is placed in prone position on a Wilson frame, with the arms tucked to the sides and with adequate padding for all pressure points. If the Wilson frame is not available, we adjust the table to place the patient in slight hip flexion, in order to open up the interlaminar space and decrease the amount of lamina needing to be removed to access the disc.

Skin Incision

The level of interest is identified on the lateral image by placing a spinal needle in alignment with the intervertebral disc to be removed (Fig. 2.1). The skin incision is centered on the spinal needle entry point and is typically 1.5–2 cm in length, parallel to the midline and about 2–5 cm lateral to it, depending on the size of the patient and the location of the disc herniation. In patients with larger body habitus, the incision has to be placed further laterally (Fig. 2.2). Also, the more central the disc

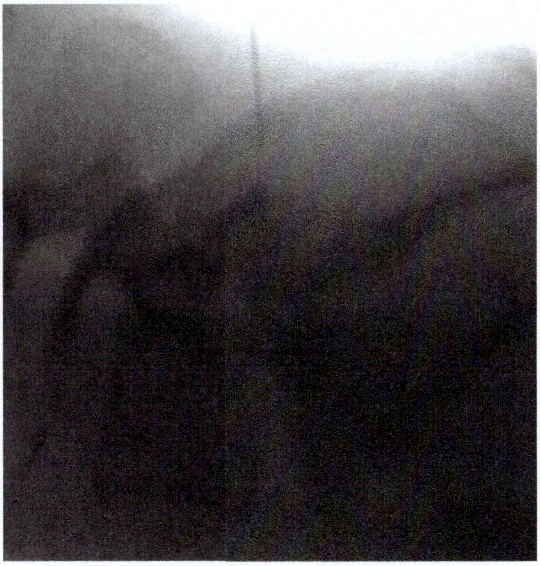

Fig. 2.1 Lateral fluoroscopic image showing the spinal needle in line with the disc of interest

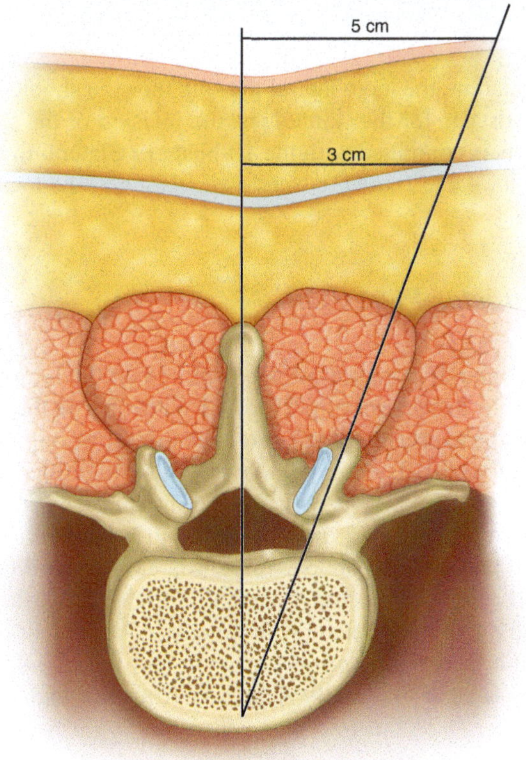

Fig. 2.2 Artist's illustration showing that the skin incision must be placed further lateral in obese patients

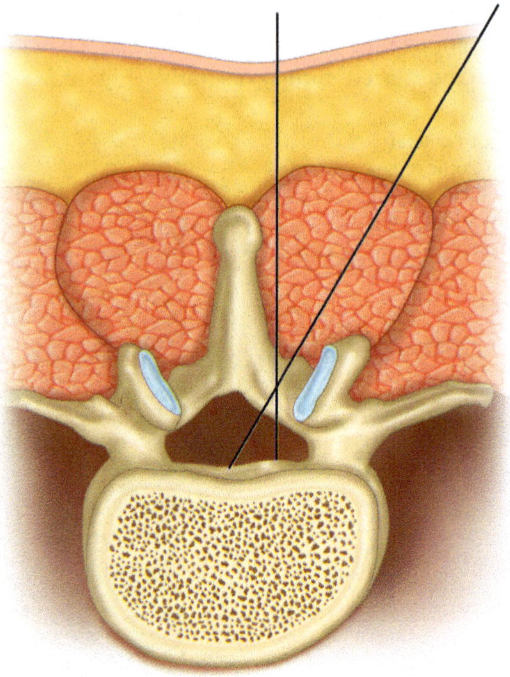

Fig. 2.3 Artist's illustration showing that the skin incision must be placed further lateral in patients with central disc herniations and closer to midline in patients with lateral recess herniations

herniation, the more lateral the skin incision should be placed (Fig. 2.3). After local hemostasis for the skin edges, the incision of the subcutaneous fat and the lumbar fascia is continued with the 10-blade in a lateral to medial direction, and maintaining the same cranial to caudal angulation as the localizing spinal needle.

Retractor Placement

The tubular retractor must be docked on the lamina of interest. The paraspinous muscle dissection is performed with one of the smaller tubular dilators. Care must be exercised not to place the dilator through the interlaminar space into the spinal canal. The bony landmark to be identified with the dilator is the junction between the spinous process and the lamina of the level of interest (e.g., the L4 lamina if the L4–5 discectomy is to be performed). This should be confirmed with lateral fluoroscopy, since it is easy to land on the level above or below, as well as AP fluoroscopy, since the dilator can pass over the spinous process and land on the contralateral lamina, particularly in obese patients. Once the junction between the spinous process and the lamina is identified, the paraspinous muscles can be gently detached from the underlying lamina with the tubular

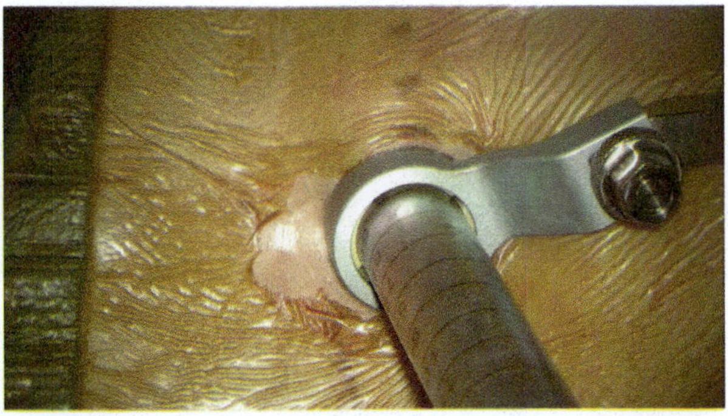

Fig. 2.4 The depth of the tubular retractor is determined by the reading the number on the side of the widest tubular dilator

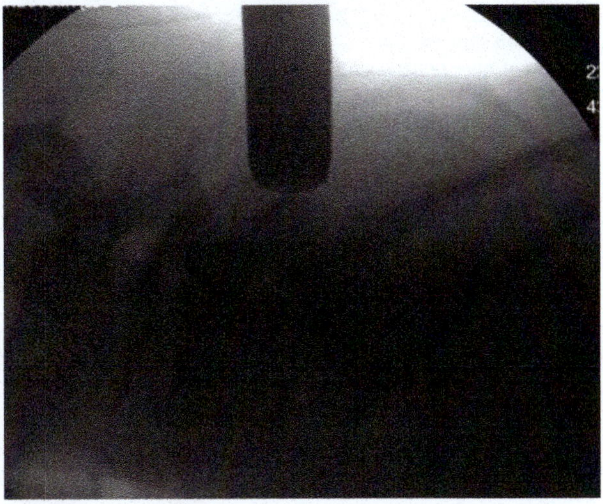

Fig. 2.5 Lateral fluoroscopic image showing the placement of the tubular retractor in line with the disc of interest

dilator, with great care not to fall in the interlaminar space and injure the spinal sac. Tubular dilators of increasing size are then used to insert the final tubular retractor of the appropriate length, as read on the side of the tubular dilators (Fig. 2.4). The correct placement of the tube, in line with the intervertebral disc of interest, is confirmed with lateral fluoroscopy (Fig. 2.5) and then the retractor is locked in place with a rigid arm (Fig. 2.6). Most surgeons prefer the 18 mm diameter retractor, although the 22 mm diameter tube can be used in larger patients. The smaller diameter retractor usually fits better on the lamina, whereas the larger diameter retractor is usually blocked by the facet complex, resulting in more space (and muscle to be removed) between the tip of the retractor and the lamina.

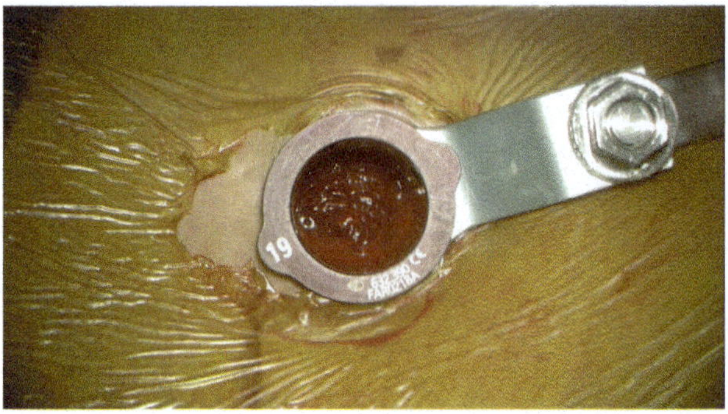

Fig. 2.6 The tubular retractor is locked in place with the rigid arm

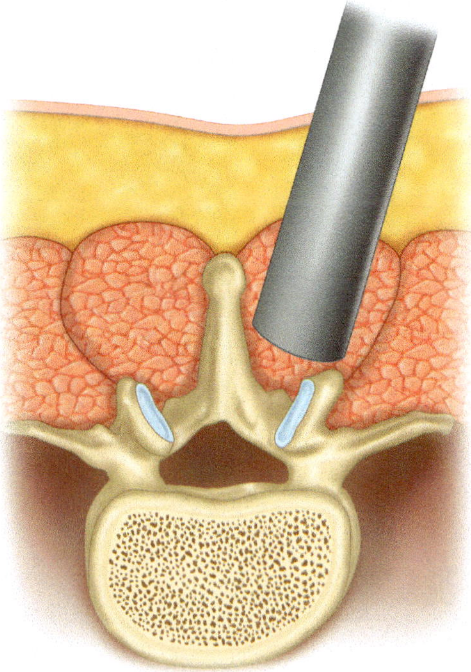

Fig. 2.7 Artist's illustration showing the amount of muscle between the tip of the retractor tube and the lamina

The next operative step is the exposure of the lamina of interest. At this point, the microscope is brought into the operative field. There is always a small amount of muscle left between the bottom of the tube and the lamina (Fig. 2.7). This muscle must be removed with the Bovie cautery and/or pituitary rongeurs, in order to expose the underlying bony anatomy. Typically, the medial edge of the tube rests against the base of the spinous process, the caudal edge of the tube is at the level of the caudal edge of the lamina, the cranial edge of the tube is just at the pars interarticularis, and the lateral edge of the tube rests on or just medial to the medial facet joint (Fig. 2.8).

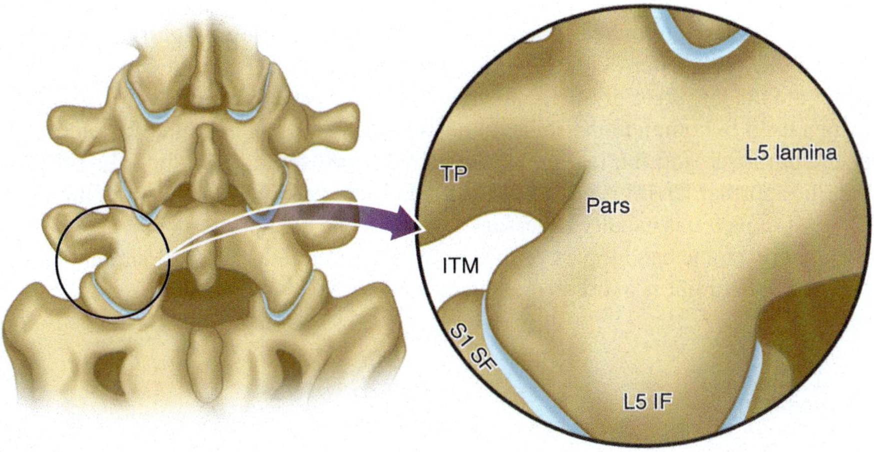

Fig. 2.8 Artist's illustration showing the typical exposure of the spinal elements as seen through the retractor tube

Laminotomy

The next operative step is the laminotomy, i.e., the removal of enough bone to allow safe exposure of the dural sac removal of the disc herniation. The bony removal is started with the high-speed drill at the caudal edge of the lamina, typically about half way between the junction with the spinous process and the medial facet. If the disc herniation is large, the laminotomy has to be extended medially to, or even under, the spinous process, in order for the spinal sac to be easier to mobilize over the herniation. The yellow ligament is encountered in the depth, underneath the lamina. The bony removal is continued cranially until the insertion of the yellow ligament is encountered (if the disc herniation is migrated cephalad) or over 3–4 mm (if the herniation is at the level or below the disc space). The removal is also extended laterally until the downward curvature of the yellow ligament is observed, suggesting that the lateral edge of the spinal sac can be exposed. Great care must be exercised not to extend the laminotomy through the pars interarticularis, which would detach the medial facet and potentially result in instability. This is always possible at L5–S1 and L4–L5, where the lamina is sufficiently wide, whereas at L3–4 and above, the lamina is too narrow and a facetectomy rather than laminotomy should be planned.

Yellow Ligament Removal

If the cranial insertion of the yellow ligament has been exposed, a small upbiting curette is flipped under the yellow ligament and followed with a Kerrison rongeur to remove the ligament in a piece-meal fashion. If the cranial insertion has not been exposed, then an 11-blade can be used to cut the yellow ligament in the direction of its fibers until a bluish hue is noticed under the microscope, signifying the closeness of the dura mater (Video 2.1). At this point, a blunt Penfield 4 can be used to penetrate the last layer of the ligament and a "pop" is usually felt. A Kerrison 2 or 3 is then used to complete the removal of the ligament. At this point, the lateral edge of the dural sac and the takeoff of the spinal nerve should be exposed; if they are not, then further lateral removal of the medial facet and yellow ligament are necessary. Moreover, it is usually necessary to remove the medial edge of the lateral facet, particularly in the caudal part of the exposure. Sometimes, a small amount of fluid from the facet joint is expressed and can mimic CSF.

Discectomy

The next operative step is the exposure and removal of the herniated disc. The epidural veins lateral to the dural sac are usually prominent and should be coagulated with the bipolar cautery on low voltage, then sharply transected. A small annulotomy with an 11 or 15-blade, lateral to the spinal sac, is usually necessary to release the herniated fragment (Video 2.4). We recommend performing this small annulotomy parallel to the edge of the spinal sac (i.e., longitudinally), just in case there was a misinterpretation of the anatomy and there is still dural sac over the disc; the longitudinal opening will still result in extravasation of CSF, but at least no nerves will be cut, as they run longitudinally in the spinal sac.

Depending on the morphology of the disc herniation, this can be identified either laterally in the lateral recess, or more medially underneath the takeoff of the spinal nerve. It is important to remember the cranio-caudal position of the herniation relative to the disc space on the MRI, in order to properly look for and remove all the disc fragments. Occasionally, the disc herniation can be adherent to the dural sac and has to be carefully detached before removal. Other times, especially in large disc herniations, a piece of endplate can be identified in the herniation. Moreover, in large disc herniations, there are usually multiple large fragments, so the surgeon should not assume that the discectomy is complete after a single large fragment removal (Video 2.1). Indirect indications that there are still some residual fragments are the lack of mobility of the spinal sac medially and lack of the typical "softness" of the spinal sac (due to an underlying disc fragment).

Regardless of the position and morphology of the herniation, a thorough inspection of the entire area with a downbiting curette or a smooth right-angle retractor is mandatory (Video 2.3). We prefer to start cranial to the disc and move the downbiting curette over the disc space and under the dural sac until reaching the caudal vertebral body, without any obstacles. The inspection is also carried out medially until reaching the midline. These landmarks are confirmed and documented with lateral (for the cranial and caudal inspection) and AP (for the medial inspection) fluoroscopic images (Fig. 2.9). Particular attention should be paid not to leave a sequestered disc fragment under the dural sac. When the decompression is complete,

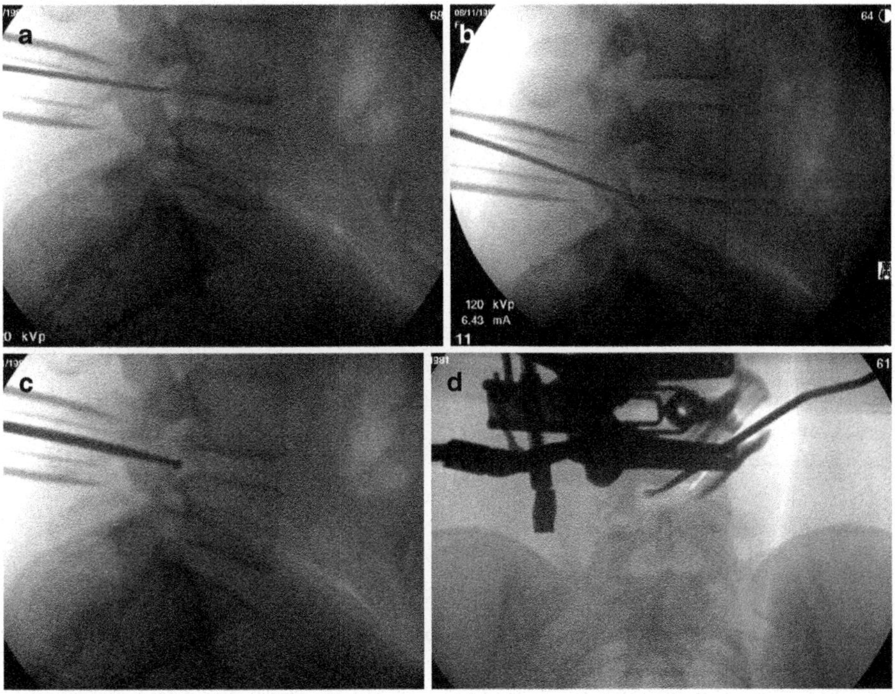

Fig. 2.9 Fluoroscopic images documenting the extent of disc removal. (**a**) and (**b**) Lateral fluoroscopic images showing the Penfield 4 as it is passed from above to below the disc without any obstacles. (**c**) When the down-biting curette is placed medially over the disc, it should be at or just above the adjacent bony edges. (**d**) The curette is maintained in the same position and an AP fluoroscopic image is taken to confirm the extent of medial decompression

the dural sac should be easy to retract medially. A Woodson tool is used at the end to follow the spinal nerve in the caudal foramen and confirm that the decompression is complete.

After the decompression, we prefer to place a Marcaine-soaked Gelfoam over the exposed dural sac for both hemostasis and postoperative pain control. Patients should be advised that they might experience a transient increase in radicular discomfort when the Marcaine effects wear off. The tubular retractor is then removed and final hemostasis of the muscle is performed with the bipolar cautery at high voltage, under microscopic visualization. Exparel can be injected in the paraspinous muscles for postoperative pain control.

Closure

The would is closed in layers with interrupted 2-0 Vycril on a UR needle for the lumbar fascia, followed by 3-0 Vycril and running subcutaneous 4-0 Monocryl for the skin (Video 2.6). In large patients, it may be impossible to close the fascia.

However, if a dural tear was inadvertently created during the surgery, we recommend a watertight fascial closure, even if that requires extending the skin incision cranially and / or caudally.

Pearls and Pitfalls

Incomplete Removal of the Disc Herniation

These patients typically present with no pain relief and the repeat MRI shows a persistent disc fragment with similar morphology as on the preoperative MRI. We prefer to re-explore and remove the remainder of the disc herniation as soon as possible, in order to avoid scar formation.

Excessive Removal of Central Disc

Traditionally, spine surgeons used to remove not only the herniated disc, but also most of the central nucleus pulposus, in order to prevent re-herniations. While it is true that the rate of re-herniations is close to zero in these patients, it is also true that a large number of them return with axial low back pain, likely due to the destabilizing effect of removing the central disc material. We therefore recommend limiting the disc removal to just the herniated part, leaving the central disc material intact [1, 2].

Calcified Discs

These are osteophytes rather than disc herniations and can be extremely difficult to remove, not only because of the size, but also because they are often adherent to the dura. In these cases, we prefer a more generous exposure laterally, attempting to allow for less spinal sac retraction until at least some of the osteophyte is removed. Unfortunately, most frequently, these osteophytes have to be removed with the high-speed drill, as the dura is detached and gently retracted medially. If the osteophytes are more centrally located, a generous laminectomy, sometimes with undercutting of the contralateral lamina, allows for easier mobilization of the dural sac over the large central osteophyte (Video 2.2). These patients should be advised preoperatively about the high incidence of dural tears.

Very Large Disc Herniations

Similar to the calcified discs described above, we recommend a more generous laminectomy laterally (to allow for less retraction of the edge of the dural sac over the disc herniation before taking out the first fragment) and medially (up to, and sometimes under, the spinous process, in order to allow for easier mobilization of the dural sac medially). If the disc herniation is very large, we recommend removing it in multiple pieces, as the dural sac will relax and become easier to mobilize with each disc fragment removed (Video 2.1).

As a general rule, if we encounter difficulty in mobilizing and removing a disc fragment, we remove more bone, either laterally, medially, cranially, or, rarely, caudally from the cranial edge of the caudal lamina), until we gain better access to the "stuck" disc fragment.

Foraminal Disc Herniations

True foraminal disc herniations can only be accessed via Parsectomy (see Chap. 4).

One option for herniations located between the lateral recess and the foramen is a contralateral skin incision and laminotomy, tilting the retractor tube to remove the yellow ligament ipsilateral to the disc herniation (and contralateral to the skin incision). This approach allows for some access to the medial aspect of the foramen, underneath the medial edge of the lateral facet [3].

Extraforaminal Disc Herniations

These herniations are rare. When they occur, the skin incision is placed 5–6 cm lateral to the midline and the tubular retractor is docked just above the junction between the caudal transverse process and the lateral facet (i.e., Wiltse approach) [4]. Following this junction cranially, the lateral aspect of the lateral facet is used as a guide to access the disc. The herniation is typically found here, with the nerve draped over its' cranial aspect. Once the herniation is removed, the nerve can be easily mobilized in its' extraforaminal course.

Migrated Disc Fragments

These types of herniations are also relatively rare.

When the fragment migrates caudally, most of the bony removal must be done on the cranial aspect of the caudal lamina (e.g., the L5 lamina for an L4–5 disc herniation) and only minimal removal of the cranial lamina is necessary (the L4 lamina in the above example). The yellow ligament removal can be started caudally, since part of the caudal lamina has already been removed, and the disc fragment is typically found in the axilla of the traversing spinal nerve (the L5 nerve in the above example) or just caudal to it.

When the fragment migrates cranially, the bony removal must also be extended cranially (e.g., the L4 lamina for an L4–5 disc herniation). Care must be exercised in these cases not to disrupt the pars interarticularis and create instability. Frequent lateral fluoroscopic images are helpful in confirming the cranial extent of the decompression.

Obese Patients

The tubular retractor is ideal for obese patients, since it provides similar deep exposure with minimal superficial morbidity [5]. However, we prefer to perform a more extensive discectomy in obese patients, including some of the central nucleus pulposus, since the increased pressure on the affected disc may represent a predisposing factor for re-herniation through the created annular defect [6].

Complications

The complications are similar to the open discectomy technique.

Durotomy

Inadvertent durotomies can occur, particularly in old disc herniations that may be adherent to the spinal sac. Due to the limited exposure, a direct repair with 4-0 Nurolon is not feasible. We prefer to temporarily cover the durotomy with a Gelfoam and patty, and complete the decompression. At the end, we place a small piece of dural substitute (e.g., DuraGuard) over the durotomy and then cover with DuraSeal [7] (Video 2.5). Most often, due to the sealing effect of the paraspinal muscles, a CSF fistula is not observed. In the few cases in which a CSF fistula does occur, we prefer placing a lumbar drain for 5–7 days, rather than re-exploring the wound.

Instability

This can result from either removing too much bone (i.e., performing a facetectomy instead of a laminotomy) or too much disc material from the central part of the disc. Unfortunately, if these patients are symptomatic (typically with axial low back pain), a fusion may become necessary. In fact, care must be exercised not to diagnose a patient who returns with axial back pain as a "recurrence" of the disc herniation, but rather suspect instability at that segment.

Re-herniation

In re-herniations, the patients experience a return of similar symptoms (i.e., leg pain) after a pain-free period. The repeat MRI typically shows a disc herniation with different morphology than the original one. The choice of performing a second (or even third) laminotomy and discectomy versus a fusion depends on patient's symptoms (i.e., increased axial low back pain would favor a fusion) as well as the amount of associated degenerative changes at that level (i.e., increased degenerative changes would also favor a fusion). In our experience, obese patients tend to have a higher rate of re-herniation and tend to do better with fusions as the second operation.

Nerve Damage

The nerve affected by the disc herniation is usually the traversing one (e.g., S1 for an L5–S1 disc herniation), since the herniation is usually paracentral. If the disc herniation is large and/or calcified, excessive medial retraction of the spinal sac may result in nerve damage, although most commonly the main symptom is persistent radiculopathy (that eventually resolves) rather than motor or sensory deficit.

Extreme care must be exercised when removing yellow ligament under the medial aspect of the lateral facet, particularly in the cranial part of the foramen, since the exiting nerve is at risk of being bitten by the Kerrison rongeur.

Massive Blood Loss

This is a rare and unfortunate complication that results from damage to the great abdominal vessels after penetration of the anterior annulus fibrosus by sharp or biting instruments. While we have not encountered this complication, it is recommended that, if vascular damage occurs, the patient should be turned immediately in supine position and abdominal exploration, preferably by a general or vascular surgeon, should be performed in order to stop the bleeding.

Literature Review

While some studies have shown no significant differences between the results of open versus tubular microdiscectomy [8–10], several "intangibles" that were not assessed in these studies make the tubular discectomy a favorite, in the authors' opinion. Many of these studies are retrospective in nature, thus leading to a selection bias. First, the angulation of the tube can be tailored to access different locations of the disc herniation, without extensive muscle dissection or bony removal. Second, the minimal scarring after tubular microdiscectomy makes subsequent interventions, if needed (e.g., for a fusion or for the treatment of recurrent herniation), easier and safer than after the open discectomy. Third, the risk of a CSF fistula after an accidental durotomy may be lower in the minimally invasive technique, due to the sealing effect of the paraspinous muscles. This was shown in a retrospective review of prospectively collected data out of Northwestern University [11]. Patients in this study were significantly less likely to require lumbar drainage for a CSF leak if they had undergone a minimally invasive decompression versus an open decompression.

A Cochrane review was able to show that minimally invasive techniques lead to a lower infection rate than their open counterparts. However, they found that the studies weren't significantly powered to detect any other changes. There are data that suggest a shorter length of stay and less blood loss when compared to open procedures, as well as improving operative times as a surgeon gets more experience in minimally invasive techniques [12–14].

The described technique can be applied for disc herniations at the L4–5 and L5–S1 levels. For herniations at the L3–4 and L2–3 levels, the lamina and pars interarticularis are too narrow and therefore the entire medial facet has to be removed in order to access the disc (Chap. 3). Foraminal disc herniations between L1 and S1 can be removed via parsectomy (Chap. 4).

Conclusion

The minimally invasive tubular microdiscectomy allows for achieving the same goals as the open discectomy, with minimal morbidity.

Addendum: Informative Letter to the Patient

The following informative letter is NOT intended to cover ALL the possible complications and scenarios. It is only intended to serve as a general guide, to improve patients' understanding of the operation.

The operation is called a microdiscectomy or laminotomy. We make a small incision (usually less than 1 in.) in the lower back, slightly off the midline to the side of the pain. The muscle tissue is gently pushed aside so we can get down to the bones of the spine. The muscles are sore, stiff, and swollen for several weeks after surgery. We then remove some of the back part of the spinal bones (laminotomy) in order to open the spinal canal. At this point an operating microscope is used to allow us to keep the incision as small as possible, yet have excellent vision so we can see what needs to be done.

The nerves are identified, and we do whatever it takes to "unpinch" them. Sometimes this means removing more bone, and sometimes it requires removal of part of the disc. We sometimes have to enter the more central part of the disc to remove loose material, which is done in order to reduce the chance of another herniation in the future (but it can still occur, and if it happens then possibly another operation will be required).

I have performed this operation many times and consider it routine. Unfortunately it is not "safe," since every procedure I do as a neurosurgeon has real risk and danger associated with it. Death from anesthesia reaction or massive blood loss is possible. Nerve damage could occur which in its worst form could mean loss of all function below the waist including movement, feeling, and bowel, bladder and sexual function. Infection could occur, and if that happens in a deep space like a disc it could take months of antibiotic treatment to cure. Fortunately, all that is very rare. There are, however, three risks, which are relatively common.

There is a 5–10% chance of dural tear and spinal fluid leakage (which is increased if there has been previous surgery with formation of scar tissue). The dura mater is a leaf that covers and protects the nerves, and is filled with fluid called CSF (cerebrospinal fluid). If the dura is torn during surgery, the fluid comes out and may get all the way to the skin. If this happens, a second operation for closure of this leakage and placement of a lumbar drain (to divert the fluid from coming out of the dural defect) is usually necessary. There is a 5–10% chance of recurrence of disc herniation, which may require a re-operation similar to the initial one, but with slightly increased risk due to scar formation. Finally, there is a 5–10% chance of painful motion between the bones developing in the future, which might lead to a fusion operation (with screws and rods).

Usually the length of hospitalization is quite brief, in fact either same day or just overnight. Unless there was a dural tear during surgery, you will be asked to get out of bed either the same day or the morning after surgery. A walking program can start within a week or two. This should be done on a level surface (not out in a field stepping in holes). Gradually the length of the walks should be increased until you are up to about 2–3 miles a day, if possible. At about 2–4 weeks there is a follow-up office visit, and at that time you can start a home back exercise program. This starts as gentle stretching and strengthening exercises, and it is normal not to be able to do all of these initially. By trial and error you will be able to develop your own custom-made exercise program by selecting those exercises that don't irritate or aggravate your condition. As the months pass, it is hoped that you will be able to do some of the exercises that you couldn't do at first. It is important, however, to try to do something each day. At about 2–6 weeks, most people can return to a light office type job, and by 12 weeks more moderate levels of activity can be resumed. Generally by about 6 months after surgery, about 80% of the improvement is reached, but full recovery (the last 20%) stretches out over a year. Generally physical therapy is not required, but patients who were injured on the job often require special consideration.

Once somebody has a bad back, they always will to some degree. Even the best operation is not a "spine transplant." Although I help many patients, I can never make anybody completely normal. Heavy manual labor and heavy lifting should be avoided. Permanent restrictions vary among individuals, but as a general guide I advise no lifting more than 40 pounds (a heavy sack of dog food) on an occasional basis, no more than 20 pounds on a frequent basis, and no excessive bending, stooping, or squatting. In addition, many patients with bad backs find it necessary to change positions frequently (i.e., after standing for a while it is necessary to sit, and viceversa).

This operation has been recommended in the belief that your condition is serious and therefore taking the risks of surgery makes sense. I believe this is a good operation that is the best choice for your particular problem. If your only affliction is pain, the decision is yours and yours alone as to whether you can live with it. While I obviously hope and believe that this operation will help you, I cannot give any guarantees or promises about results. It is possible that you could be the same or even worse. Furthermore, my general recommendation is to "live with it" if possible and avoid the risks and uncertainties of surgery. Nevertheless I am offering my surgical services in an attempt to help you, but the decision to proceed is up to you.

References

1. Lee SH, Bae JS. Comparison of clinical and radiological outcomes after automated open lumbar discectomy and conventional microdiscectomy: a prospective randomized trial. Int J Clin Exp Med. 2015;8:12135–48.
2. Soliman J, et al. Limited microdiscectomy for lumbar disk herniation: a retrospective long-term outcome analysis. J Spinal Disord Tech. 2014;27:E8–E13. https://doi.org/10.1097/BSD.0b013e31828da8f1.
3. Berra LV, et al. Contralateral approach for far lateral lumbar disc herniations: a modified technique and outcome analysis of nine patients. Spine. 2010;35:709–13. https://doi.org/10.1097/BRS.0b013e3181bac710.
4. T Siu TL, Lin K. Direct tubular lumbar microdiscectomy for far lateral disc herniation: a modified approach. Orthop Surg. 2016;8:301–8. https://doi.org/10.1111/os.12263.
5. Yoo MW, Hyun SJ, Kim KJ, Jahng TA, Kim HJ. Does obesity make an influence on surgical outcomes following lumbar microdiscectomy? Korean J Spine. 2014;11:68–73. https://doi.org/10.14245/kjs.2014.11.2.68.
6. Meredith DS, Huang RC, Nguyen J, Lyman S. Obesity increases the risk of recurrent herniated nucleus pulposus after lumbar microdiscectomy. Spine J. 2010;10:575–80. https://doi.org/10.1016/j.spinee.2010.02.021.
7. Kogias E, et al. Incidental durotomy in open vs. tubular revision microdiscectomy: a retrospective controlled study on incidence, management and outcome. Clin Spine Surg. 2016. https://doi.org/10.1097/bsd.0000000000000279.
8. Rasouli MR, Rahimi-Movaghar V, Shokraneh F, Moradi-Lakeh M, Chou R. Minimally invasive discectomy versus microdiscectomy/open discectomy for symptomatic lumbar disc herniation. Cochrane Database Syst Rev. 2014:CD010328. https://doi.org/10.1002/14651858.CD010328.pub2.
9. Kamper SJ, et al. Minimally invasive surgery for lumbar disc herniation: a systematic review and meta-analysis. Eur Spine J. 2014;23:1021–43. https://doi.org/10.1007/s00586-013-3161-2.
10. Lau D, Han SJ, Lee JG, Lu DC, Chou D. Minimally invasive compared to open microdiscectomy for lumbar disc herniation. J Clin Neurosci. 2011;18:81–4. https://doi.org/10.1016/j.jocn.2010.04.040.

11. Wong AP, et al. Comparison of symptomatic cerebral spinal fluid leak between patients undergoing minimally invasive versus open lumbar foraminotomy, discectomy, or laminectomy. World Neurosurg. 2014;81:634–40. https://doi.org/10.1016/j.wneu.2013.11.012.
12. Ahn J, et al. Minimally invasive lumbar decompression-the surgical learning curve. Spine J. 2016;16:909–16. https://doi.org/10.1016/j.spinee.2015.07.455.
13. Johans SJ, Amin BY, Mummaneni PV. Minimally invasive lumbar decompression for lumbar stenosis: review of clinical outcomes and cost effectiveness. J Neurosurg Sci. 2015;59:37–45.
14. Phan K, Mobbs RJ. Minimally invasive versus open laminectomy for lumbar stenosis: a systematic review and meta-analysis. Spine. 2016;41:E91–E100. https://doi.org/10.1097/brs.0000000000001161.

Chapter 3
Facetectomy

Anthony Digiorgio, Malcolm Daniel Eggart, Adriana Constantinescu, Jason Wilson, and Gabriel Tender

Introduction

Minimally invasive lumbar tubular facetectomy can be regarded as a variant of the microdiscectomy that applies to the L3–4 and L2–3 levels, where the narrow shape of the lamina and pars interarticularis forces the surgeon to remove the medial facet in order to access the disc. The L1–2 level can also be approached this way if the disc herniation is not central, since the conus medullaris typically ends at this level and therefore manipulation of the spinal sac must be minimized.

Electronic Supplementary Material The online version of this chapter https://doi.org/10.1007/978-3-319-71943-6_3. contains supplementary material, which is available to authorized users.

A. Digiorgio
Department of Neurosurgery, Louisiana State University Health Sciences Center, New Orleans, LA, USA
e-mail: Adigi2@lsuhsc.edu

M.D. Eggart
MUSC Health Neurosciences at Tidelands Health, Murrells Inlet, SC, USA

A. Constantinescu
Universitatea de Medicina si Farmacie, Craiova, Romania

J. Wilson
Department of Neurosurgery, Louisiana State University Health Sciences Center, New Orleans, LA, USA
e-mail: Jwils8@lsuhsc.edu

G. Tender (✉)
Louisiana State University, New Orleans, LA, USA

G. Tender (ed.), *Minimally Invasive Spine Surgery Techniques*,
https://doi.org/10.1007/978-3-319-71943-6_3

Indications

The indications for lumbar minimally invasive facetectomy are the same as for the open facetectomy—unilateral lumbar stenosis with compression of a spinal nerve and resultant radiculopathy, due to one or more of the following:

- herniated nucleus pulposus
- facet or yellow ligament hypertrophy
- synovial cysts or other space occupying lesions.

Most surgeons recommend a short course of conservative treatment prior to surgical intervention, with the caveat that delaying the nerve decompression for more than 6 months from the onset of symptoms may result in chronic pain and/or persistent sensory/motor deficits, despite removal of the herniated disc.

Contraindications

There are no absolute contraindications for this technique.

A relative contraindication is a recurrent disc herniation that was initially treated by an open discectomy. In these cases, the same skin incision should be used. If the initial herniation was treated in a minimally invasive fashion, it should also be re-explored through the same incision, with a tubular retractor.

Another relative contraindication is morbid obesity, when the distance between the skin surface and the lamina is over 100 mm (the longest typical tubular retractor). However, since the fat is depressible, we have used this technique in many morbidly obese patients without having to convert to an open procedure.

Surgical Technique

The following operative steps are described:

- positioning
- skin incision
- retractor placement
- laminotomy
- yellow ligament removal
- discectomy
- closure

Positioning

The patient is placed in prone position on a Wilson frame, with the arms tucked to the sides and with adequate padding for all pressure points. If the Wilson frame is not available, we adjust the table to place the patient in slight hip flexion, in order to open up the interlaminar space and decrease the amount of lamina needing to be removed to access the disc.

Skin Incision

The level of interest is identified on the lateral image by placing a spinal needle in alignment with the intervertebral disc to be removed. The skin incision is centered on the spinal needle entry point, and is typically 1.5 cm in length, parallel to the midline and about 2–3 cm lateral to it. In patients with larger body habitus, the incision has to be placed further laterally. Also, the more central the disc herniation, the more lateral the skin incision should be placed. However, since the spinal canal is much more narrow at these levels than at the L4–5 and L5–S1, the skin incision is rarely more than 3 cm lateral to the midline. After local hemostasis for the skin edges, the incision of the subcutaneous fat and the lumbar fascia is continued with the 10-blade in a lateral to medial direction, and maintaining the same angulation as the localizing spinal needle.

Retractor Placement

The first operative step is placement of the tubular retractor over the lamina of interest. The paraspinous muscle dissection is performed with one of the smaller tubular dilators. Care must be exercised not to place the dilator through the interlaminar space into the spinal canal. The bony landmark to be identified with the dilator is the junction between the spinous process and the lamina of the level of interest (e.g., the L2 lamina if the L2–3 discectomy is to be performed). This should be confirmed with lateral fluoroscopy, since it is easy to land on the level above or below, as well as AP fluoroscopy, since the dilator can pass over the spinous process and land on the contralateral lamina, particularly in large patients. Once the junction between the spinous process and the lamina is identified, the paraspinous muscles can be gently detached from the underlying lamina with the tubular dilator, with great care not to fall in the interlaminal space and injure the spinal sac. The tubular dilators of increasing size are then used to insert the final tubular retractor of the appropriate length, as read on the side of the tubular dilators. The correct placement of the tube, in line with the intervertebral disc of interest, is confirmed with lateral fluoroscopy and then the retractor is locked in place with a rigid arm. Most surgeons prefer the 18 mm diameter retractor, although the 22 mm diameter tube can be used in larger patients. The smaller diameter retractor usually fits better on the lamina, whereas the larger diameter retractor is usually blocked by the facet complex, resulting in more space (and muscle to be removed) between the tip of the retractor and the lamina.

The next operative step is the exposure of the lamina of interest. At this point, the microscope is brought into the operative field. There is always a small amount of muscle left between the bottom of the tube and the lamina. This muscle must be removed with the Bovie cautery and/or pituitary rongeurs, in order to expose the underlying bony anatomy. Typically, due to the decreased width of the lamina, the exposure through the 18 mm diameter tube allows for identification of the lamina, pars interarticularis, and medial and lateral facets, in a single field.

Facetectomy

The next operative step is the facetectomy. The bony removal is started with the high-speed drill at the caudal edge of the lamina, typically at the junction between the spinous process and the lamina. The bony removal inevitably extends laterally into the pars interarticularis, thus dislodging the medial facet (Video 3.1). The pars can be removed up to the caudal edge of the pedicle, thus allowing for exposure (and decompression, if necessary) of the exiting nerve root (e.g., L2 nerve when exposing the L2–3 disc).

Yellow Ligament Removal

The next operative step is the yellow ligament removal. Since its' cranial insertion has already been exposed, a small up-biting curette is flipped under the yellow ligament and followed with a Kerrison rongeour to remove the ligament in a piece-meal fashion. At this point, the lateral edge of the dural sac and the takeoff of the spinal nerve are exposed. It is usually necessary to also remove the medial edge of the lateral facet, particularly in the caudal part of the exposure. The smooth, shiny articular surface of the lateral facet can be seen in the field.

Discectomy

The next operative step is the exposure and removal of the herniated disc. The epidural veins lateral to the dural sac are usually prominent and should be coagulated with the bipolar cautery on low voltage, then sharply transected. A small annulotomy with an

11-blade, lateral to the spinal sac, is usually necessary to release the herniated fragment. Depending on the morphology of the disc herniation, this can be identified either laterally in the lateral recess, or more medially underneath the takeoff of the spinal nerve. It is important to remember the cranio-caudal position of the herniation relative to the disc space on the MRI, in order to properly look for and remove all the disc fragments. Occasionally, the disc herniation can be adherent to the dural sac and has to be carefully detached before removal. Other times, especially in large disc herniations, a piece of endplate can be identified in the herniation. Regardless of the position and morphology of the herniation, a thorough inspection of the entire area with a down-biting curette or a smooth right-angle retractor is mandatory. We prefer to start cranial to the disc and move the down-biting curette over the disc space and under the dural sac until reaching the caudal vertebral body, without any obstacles. The inspection is also carried out medially until reaching the midline. These landmarks are confirmed and documented with lateral (for the cranial and caudal inspection) and AP (for the medial inspection) fluoroscopic images. Particular attention should be paid not to leave a sequestered disc fragment under the dural sac. When the decompression is complete, the dural sac should be easy to retract medially. A Woodson tool is used at the end to follow the spinal nerve in the caudal foramen and confirm that the decompression is complete.

After the decompression, we prefer to place a Marcaine-soaked Gelfoam over the exposed dural sac for both hemostasis and postoperative pain control. Patients should be advised that they may experience a transient increase in radicular discomfort when the Marcaine effects wear off. The tubular retractor is then removed and final hemostasis of the muscle is performed with the bipolar cautery at high voltage, under microscopic visualization. Exparel can be injected in the paraspinous muscles for postoperative pain control.

Closure

The would is closed in layers with interrupted 2-0 Vycril on a UR needle for the lumbar fascia, followed by 3-0 Vycril and running subcutaneous 4-0 Monocryl for the skin. In large patients, it may be impossible to close the fascia. However, if a dural tear was inadvertently created during the surgery, we recommend a watertight fascial closure, even if that requires extending the skin incision cranially and/or caudally.

Pearls and Pitfalls

Incomplete Removal of the Disc Herniation

These patients typically present with no pain relief and the repeat MRI shows a persistent disc fragment with similar morphology as on the preoperative MRI. We prefer to re-explore and remove the remainder of the disc herniation as soon as possible, in order to avoid extensive scar formation.

Excessive Removal of Central Disc

Traditionally, spine surgeons used to remove not only the herniated disc, but also most of the central nucleus pulposus, in order to prevent re-herniations. While it is true that re-herniations are close to zero in these patients, it is also true that a large number of them return with axial low back pain, likely due to the destabilizing effect of removing the central disc material. We therefore recommend limiting the disc removal to just the herniated part, leaving the central disc material intact.

Calcified Discs

These are osteophytes rather than disc herniations and can be extremely difficult to remove, not only because of the size, but also because they are often adherent to the dura. In these cases, we prefer a more generous exposure laterally, attempting to allow for less spinal sac retraction until at least some of the osteophyte is removed. Unfortunately, most frequently, these osteophytes have to be removed with the high-speed drill, as the dura is detached and gently retracted medially. If the osteophytes are more centrally located, a generous laminectomy, sometimes with undercutting of the contralateral lamina, allows for easier mobilization of the dural sac over the large central osteophyte. These patients should be advised preoperatively about the high incidence of dural tears.

Very Large Disc Herniations

Similar to the calcified discs described above, we recommend a more generous laminectomy laterally (to allow for less retraction of the edge of the dural sac over the disc herniation before taking out the first fragment) and medially (up to, and sometimes under, the spinous process, in order to allow for easier mobilization of the dural sac medially). If the disc herniation is very large, we recommend removing it in multiple pieces, as the dural sac will relax and become easier to mobilize with each disc fragment removed.

Foraminal Disc Herniations

Foraminal herniations are easily accessed after medial facetectomy, since the pars interarticularis as well as the tip of the lateral facet can be removed, thus exposing the entire foraminal (as well as extraforaminal) aspect of the disc.

Extraforaminal Disc Herniations

These herniations are rare. When they occur, the skin incision is placed 5–6 cm lateral to the midline and the tubular retractor is docked just above the junction between the caudal transverse process and the lateral facet (i.e., Wiltse approach) [1]. Following this junction cranially, the lateral aspect of the lateral facet is used as a guide to access the disc. The herniation is typically found here, with the nerve draped over its' cranial aspect. Once the herniation is removed, the nerve can be easily mobilized in its' extraforaminal course.

Obese Patients

The tubular retractor is ideal for obese patients, since it provides similar deep exposure with minimal superficial morbidity. However, we prefer to perform a more extensive discectomy in obese patients, including some of the central nucleus pulposus, since the increased pressure on the affected disc may represent a predisposing factor for re-herniation through the created annular defect [2].

Removal of Foreign Bodies

We have successfully removed bullet fragments from the spinal canal with excellent results (Videos 3.2 and 3.3). The main advantage of the minimally invasive approach is that the paraspinous muscles offer a sealing effect and therefore the risk of CSF fistula is minimized.

Complications

The complications are similar to the open discectomy technique.

Durotomy

Inadvertent durotomies can occur, particularly in old disc herniations that may be adherent to the spinal sac. Due to the limited exposure, a direct repair with 4-0 Nurolon is not feasible. We prefer to temporarily cover the durotomy with a Gelfoam and patty, and complete the decompression. At the end, we place a small piece of DuraGuard or DuraMatrix over the durotomy and then cover with DuraSeal [3]. Most often, due to the sealing effect of the muscle, a CSF fistula is not observed. In the few cases in which a CSF fistula does occur, we prefer placing a lumbar drain for 5–7 days, rather than re-exploring the wound.

Instability

This technique involves unilateral removal of the articulating facets and is destabilizing, particularly in rotation [4–8]. The patient should be advised that he/she may experience increased axial pain, which may require a fusion of that level at a later time.

If a fusion is necessary, we recommend the minimally invasive lateral transpsoas approach, which allows for placement of a large interbody graft and avoids the scar from the previous posterior approach.

Re-herniation

In re-herniations, the patients experience a return of similar symptoms (i.e., leg pain) after a pain-free period. The repeat MRI typically shows a disc herniation with different morphology than the original one. The choice of performing a second laminotomy and discectomy versus a fusion depends on patient's symptoms (i.e., increased axial low back pain would favor a fusion) as well as the amount of associated degenerative changes at that level (i.e., increased degenerative changes would also favor a fusion). In our experience, obese patients tend to have a higher rate of re-herniation and tend to do better with fusions as the second operation.

Literature Review

The majority of cases involving medial facetectomy are in the context of a fusion procedure and the recent literature reflects this. However, there have been some studies reflecting the biomechanics of facetectomy, as well as its use in a patient population. The biomechanical results are mixed. Natarajan et al. showed that both unilateral & bilateral facetectomy increase torsional motion in the lumbar spine [5]. Lee & Teo showed that a laminectomy with bilateral facetectomy at L2–3 does increase motion and annulus stress with rotation, flexion and extension, but not lateral bending. However, they did not find this with unilateral facetectomy [4].

The complete medial facetectomy to access disc herniations was initially advocated [9, 10], due to the excellent results in terms of resolution of radiculopathy and relatively low incidence of clinically significant segmental instability. A series by Garrido & Connaughton in 1991 showed that, of 41 patients undergoing a facetectomy for decompression, only one required an eventual fusion with an average follow up of 22 months [9]. However, over time, it became clear that complete removal of the medial facet is destabilizing [4–8]. Nonetheless, we continue to use the facetectomy technique at L2–3 and L3–4 without a fusion, as long as the patient understands and consents to the risks of instability.

Conclusion

The tubular minimally invasive facetectomy at L3–4 and above allows for achieving the same goals as the open facetectomy, with minimal morbidity.

References

1. T Siu TL, Lin K. Direct tubular lumbar microdiscectomy for far lateral disc herniation: a modified approach. Orthop Surg. 2016;8:301–8. https://doi.org/10.1111/os.12263.
2. Meredith DS, Huang RC, Nguyen J, Lyman S. Obesity increases the risk of recurrent herniated nucleus pulposus after lumbar microdiscectomy. Spine J. 2010;10:575–80. https://doi.org/10.1016/j.spinee.2010.02.021.
3. Kogias E, et al. Incidental durotomy in open vs. tubular revision microdiscectomy: a retrospective controlled study on incidence, management and outcome. Clin Spine Surg. 2016. doi:https://doi.org/10.1097/bsd.0000000000000279.
4. Lee KK, Teo EC. Effects of laminectomy and facetectomy on the stability of the lumbar motion segment. Med Eng Phys. 2004;26:183–92. https://doi.org/10.1016/j.medengphy.2003.11.006.
5. Natarajan RN, Andersson GB, Patwardhan AG, Andriacchi TP. Study on effect of graded facetectomy on change in lumbar motion segment torsional flexibility using three-dimensional continuum contact representation for facet joints. J Biomech Eng. 1999;121:215–21.
6. Smith ZA, et al. Biomechanical effects of a unilateral approach to minimally invasive lumbar decompression. PLoS one. 2014;9:e92611. https://doi.org/10.1371/journal.pone.0092611.
7. Teo EC, Lee KK, Qiu TX, Ng HW, Yang K. The biomechanics of lumbar graded facetectomy under anterior-shear load. IEEE Trans Biomed Eng. 2004;51:443–9. https://doi.org/10.1109/tbme.2003.821009.
8. Zander T, Rohlmann A, Klockner C, Bergmann G. Influence of graded facetectomy and laminectomy on spinal biomechanics. Eur Spine J. 2003;12:427–34. https://doi.org/10.1007/s00586-003-0540-0.
9. Garrido E, Connaughton PN. Unilateral facetectomy approach for lateral lumbar disc herniation. J Neurosurg. 1991;74:754–6. https://doi.org/10.3171/jns.1991.74.5.0754.
10. Frizzell RT, Hadley MN. Lumbar microdiscectomy with medial facetectomy. Techniques and analysis of results. Neurosurg Clin N Am. 1993;4:109–15.

Chapter 4
Parsectomy

Rand Voorhies, Gabriel Tender, Clifford Crutcher, and Anthony Digiorgio

Introduction

Lumbar tubular parsectomy is an approach similar to the microdiscectomy, which can be applied to any lumbar or even thoracic level. The parsectomy can be employed when the entire length of a specific spinal nerve needs to be decompressed.

Indications

The indication for parsectomy is foraminal stenosis with resultant radiculopathy. This is usually due to foraminal disc herniations, but occasionally the foraminal stenosis is due to a combination of disc protrusion, yellow ligament hypertrophy, facet hypertrophy, and even spondylolisthesis (in this last case, a fusion at the respective level is usually indicated, instead of a simple parsectomy). Biomechanical analysis has demonstrated that unilateral parsectomy does not significantly destabilize the spine.

Electronic Supplementary Material The online version of this chapter https://doi.org/10.1007/978-3-319-71943-6_4. contains supplementary material, which is available to authorized users.

R. Voorhies
Southern Brain and Spine, Metairie, LA, USA
e-mail: voorhies@sbsdocs.net

G. Tender (✉)
Louisiana State University, New Orleans, LA, USA

C. Crutcher • A. Digiorgio
Department of Neurosurgery, Louisiana State University Health Sciences Center, New Orleans, LA, USA
e-mail: ccrutc@lsuhsc.edu; Adigi2@lsuhsc.edu

G. Tender (ed.), *Minimally Invasive Spine Surgery Techniques*,
https://doi.org/10.1007/978-3-319-71943-6_4

Contraindications

A specific contraindication is the existence of a previous laminotomy. In this case, the parsectomy would lead to detachment of the medial facet, and thus potential instability.

Surgical Anatomy

The pars interarticularis is the connecting part between the superior and inferior facet of any given spinal level (Fig. 4.1). The pars is located just caudal to the corresponding pedicle and overlies the trajectory of the nerve exiting at the respective level (Fig. 4.2). The pars is widest at L5 and gets narrower with each level cranial to it (Fig. 4.3). If only the pars interarticularis is removed, the corresponding lamina remains anchored to the inferior facet and its joint, and therefore the level is not destabilized.

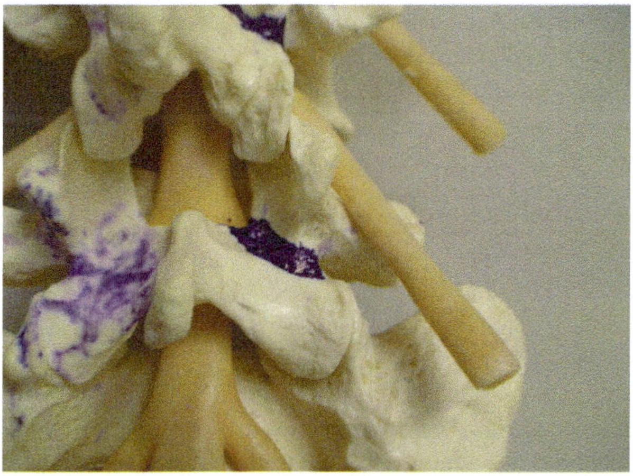

Fig. 4.1 Posterior view of the right L5 pars interarticularis in a spine model, illustrating its slightly oblique direction

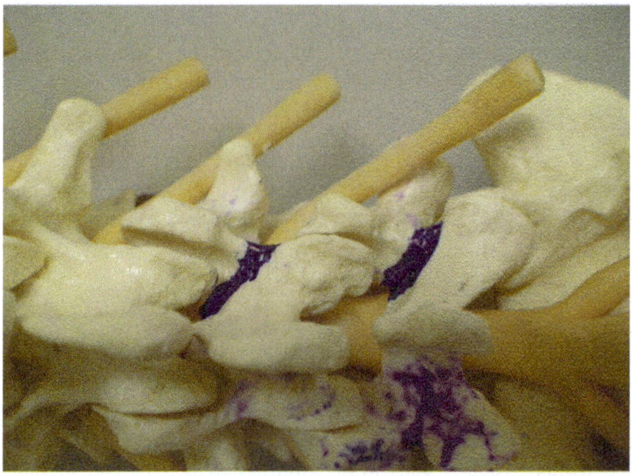

Fig. 4.2 Posterior view of the right L3, L4, and L5 pars interarticularis in a spine model, illustrating the progressive decrease in width from caudal to cranial

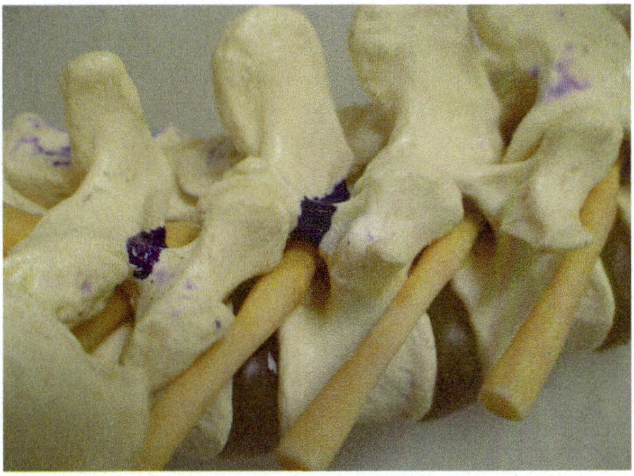

Fig. 4.3 Oblique view of the right L5 pars interarticularis in a spine model, illustrating the report between the pars, the corresponding pedicle, and the spinal nerve

Surgical Technique

The following operative steps are described:

- positioning
- skin incision
- retractor placement
- parsectomy
- discectomy
- closure

Positioning

The patient is placed in prone position on a Wilson frame, with the arms tucked to the sides and with adequate padding for all pressure points. If the Wilson frame is not available, we adjust the table to place the patient in slight hip flexion, in order to open up the interlaminar space and decrease the amount of lamina needing to be removed to access the disc.

Skin Incision

The level of interest is identified on the lateral image by placing a spinal needle in alignment with the pars interarticularis of interest, which is located just caudal to the corresponding pedicle (Fig. 4.1). The skin incision is centered on the spinal needle entry point, and is typically 1.5–2 cm in length, parallel to the midline and about 2–3 cm lateral to it. After local hemostasis for the skin edges, the incision of the subcutaneous fat and the lumbar fascia is continued with the 10-blade in a straight-down fashion (no or minimal lateral to medial angulation), but maintaining the same cranial to caudal angulation as the localizing spinal needle.

Retractor Placement

The tubular retractor must be docked on the pars interarticularis of interest. The paraspinous muscle dissection is performed with one of the smaller tubular dilators in a straight-down fashion, in a longitudinal plane, parallel to the spinous process. Care must be exercised not to place the dilator through the interlaminar space into the spinal canal. The bony landmark to be identified with the dilator is the "valley between the two hills" (e.g., the L4 pars will be the "valley" between the two "hills" of the L3–4 and L4–5 facets). On lateral fluoroscopy, this should be just below the corresponding pedicle (the L4 pedicle, in our example). On AP fluoroscopy, the dilator should be between the two rings of the cranial and caudal pedicles (L4 and L5 in our example). Once the pars interarticularis is identified by direct palpation as well as fluoroscopy, the paraspinous muscles can be gently detached from the underlying bone with the tubular dilator, and then tubular dilators of increasing size are used to insert the final tubular retractor of the appropriate length, as read on the side of the largest tubular dilator. The correct placement of the tube, in line with the pars interarticularis of interest, is confirmed with lateral fluoroscopy and then the retractor is locked in place with a rigid arm. Most surgeons prefer the 18 mm diameter retractor, although the 22 mm diameter tube can be used in larger patients.

The next operative step is the exposure of the pars interarticularis of interest. At this point, the microscope is brought into the operative field. There is always a small amount of muscle left between the bottom of the tube and the pars interarticularis, since the edges of the tube rest on the bulkier facet joints above and below. Once the small amount of muscle is removed, the pars is easily identified not only by its anatomic location, but also by the smooth, shiny, curved appearance of its lateral aspect.

Parsectomy

The next operative step is the removal of the pars interarticularis, to allow safe exposure of the underlying nerve and possibly removal of a disc herniation (Video 4.1). The bony removal is started with the high-speed drill at the lateral edge of the pars interarticularis, with great care not to violate the corresponding pedicle; this can be easily done by taking a lateral fluoroscopic image, marking the caudal edge of the pedicle on the pars interarticularis with the Bovie or the high-speed drill, and staying caudal to that mark with the bony removal. Subsequent lateral images can be taken as the drill goes deeper and deeper into the pars interarticularis. Occasionally, the lumbar artery, located just lateral to the pars interarticularis in the soft tissues, may be violated with the high-speed drill, but the bleeding can be easily identified and controlled with the bipolar cautery.

The pars interarticularis can be quite thick, particularly in patients with advanced degeneration and bony hypertrophy, and the novice surgeon may get lost because of the large amount of bone that needs to be removed to reach the yellow ligament and underlying nerve. We recommend taking multiple lateral images during this operative step, confirming that the foramen has not been reached yet. Alternatively, the lateral images may show that the surgeon has steered cranially and is now in the pedicle rather than towards the foramen. In this case, more caudal bony removal is performed.

Eventually, soft tissue is encountered, and that marks the access to the foramen. The width of the parsectomy (in cranio-caudal direction) is typically 4–6 mm, sufficient to expose the underlying nerve and remove any foraminal disc herniation, if present. The parsectomy is continued medially; however, the surgeon must be mindful that the spinal canal will be encountered, and therefore the direction of the drill bit must be changed to a more lateral to medial direction, in order to not damage the underlying dura. There is no yellow ligament at this level, which makes drilling even more dangerous than, for example, during a laminotomy. The pars interarticularis has a slightly oblique direction (Fig. 4.1) and thus drilling off the pars must follow this direction. Once the edge of the spinal sac is encountered medially, the origin of the exiting spinal nerve can be easily identified just medial to the corresponding pedicle. The nerve can be now followed from medial to lateral, all the way out to the soft tissues, although in its' foraminal portion it is often covered by yellow ligament, and at the junction with its' extraforaminal portion it is crossed by a small artery (the "arcade of Dunsker"). Occasionally, in patients with collapsed discs, the tip of the lateral facet has to be removed in order to achieve a good neural decompression.

At L5, and occasionally at L4, the pars interarticularis is wide enough that only a partial removal may be sufficient (aka "fenestration"). The location of this partial pars interarticularis removal (i.e., medial, central, or lateral) can be tailored to the specific area of stenosis and/or disc herniation and may offer increased postoperative stability.

Discectomy

A foraminal disc herniation can be easily accessed, if present, after the parsectomy is complete. The disc fragments are typically located caudal to the nerve, pushing it cranially against the pedicle. This approach is not designed to remove the normally located part of the disc, since full access to the annulus fibrosus would require extension of the parsectomy into the caudal joint, which may result in instability (in fact, extension of the parsectomy into the caudal facet joint would mimic the exposure for an MI TLIF).

Closure

The would is closed in layers with interrupted 2-0 Vycril on a UR needle for the lumbar fascia, followed by 3-0 Vycril and running subcutaneous 4-0 Monocryl for the skin. In large patients, it may be impossible to close the fascia. However, if a dural tear was inadvertently created during the surgery, we recommend a watertight fascial closure, even if that requires extending the skin incision cranially and/or caudally.

Pearls and Pitfalls

The bony removal can also be done from medial to lateral, by starting the drilling at the medial edge of the pars and following the dural sac to its edge and then continuing to drill the pars laterally, over the exiting nerve and just caudal to the corresponding pedicle. With either exposure, the surgeon must be mindful of the almost perpendicular change in direction from the spinal canal to the lateral pars, and adjust the position of the drill accordingly.

Another trick to decrease bleeding as well as the risk of an incidental durotomy is to use a diamond drill bit. Disadvantages of this technique include a slower progression of the drilling and the need for extensive irrigation, since the diamond burr gets hot very quickly.

Complications

The complications are relatively rare.

Durotomy

Inadvertent durotomies can occur, particularly if the direction of the drill bit is not adjusted to stay perpendicular to the dural surface, when switching from the lateral pars to the part covering the spinal canal. Due to the limited exposure, a direct repair with 4-0 Nurolon is not feasible. We prefer to temporarily cover the durotomy with a Gelfoam and patty, and complete the decompression. At the end, we place a small piece of DuraGuard or DuraMatrix over the durotomy and then cover with DuraSeal [1]. Most often, due to the sealing effect of the paraspinal muscles, a CSF fistula is not observed. In the few cases in which a CSF fistula does occur, we prefer placing a lumbar drain for 5–7 days, rather than re-exploring the wound.

Instability

This can result from removing too much bone (i.e., extending the parsectomy into the caudal joint). Unfortunately, if these patients are symptomatic (typically with axial low back pain), a fusion may become necessary.

Nerve Damage

Damage to the underlying, exiting spinal nerve is rare, but when it occurs, it can result in more pain than usual, since the exposed dorsal root ganglia contains first-order neurons. Careful drilling and avoidance of sharp objects after the bone is removed may help prevent this complication.

Literature Review

This procedure is much less common than the laminotomy and microdiscectomy, hence the published literature is scarce.

Di Lorenzo [2] first described the pars interarticularis fenestration for removal of foraminal disc herniations.

A biomechanical study [3] showed that unilateral parsectomy is not destabilizing, since the caudal facet remains connected via the ipsilateral joint to the caudal segment.

A retrospective clinical study [4] showed that parsectomy offered good pain relief in a select group of patients.

Conclusion

Minimally invasive unilateral removal of the pars interarticularis provides excellent neural decompression in patients with foraminal stenosis, regardless of the etiology, and is not destabilizing.

References

1. Kogias E, et al. Incidental durotomy in open vs. tubular revision microdiscectomy: a retrospective controlled study on incidence, management and outcome. Clin Spine Surg. 2016. https://doi.org/10.1097/bsd.0000000000000279.

2. Di Lorenzo N, et al. Pars interarticularis fenestration in the treatment of foraminal lumbar disc herniation: a further surgical approach. Neurosurgery. 1998;42:87–9; discussion 89-90.
3. Tender GC, Baratta RV, Voorhies RM. Unilateral removal of pars interarticularis. J Neurosurg Spine. 2005;2:279–88. https://doi.org/10.3171/spi.2005.2.3.0279.
4. Tender GC, Kutz S, Baratta R, Voorhies RM. Unilateral progressive alterations in the lumbar spine: a biomechanical study. J Neurosurg Spine. 2005;2:298–302. https://doi.org/10.3171/spi.2005.2.3.0298.

Chapter 5
Laminectomy

Zachary A. Medress, Yi-Ren Chen, Ian Connolly, John Ratliff, and Atman Desai

Introduction

Spinal stenosis is the most common indication for surgery in the lumbar spine [1]. A minimally invasive approach through a tubular retractor provides direct surgical access to decompress the central canal and lateral recess in patients with evidence of central stenosis due to broad based disc bulges, ligamentum flavum hypertrophy, and facet arthropathy. Benefits of a minimally invasive laminectomy include smaller incision, less muscular disruption and pain, reduced blood loss and rate of blood transfusion, reduced rate of blood transfusion, preservation of components of the midline tension band including interspinous ligaments, spinous process, supraspinous ligament.

Indications

Patients suited for a MIS laminectomy include those that present with neurogenic claudication from central canal stenosis and/or lumbar radiculopathy from lateral recess stenosis. Unilateral or bilateral lateral recess stenosis from ligamentum flavum hypertrophy, facet arthropathy should be visualized on MRI at a level that corresponds with the patient's symptoms in the absence of spondylolisthesis, deformity, or evidence of motion on lumbar flexion-extension X-rays.

Electronic Supplementary Material The online version of this chapter https://doi.org/10.1007/978-3-319-71943-6_5. contains supplementary material, which is available to authorized users.

Z.A. Medress • Y.-R. Chen • I. Connolly • J. Ratliff (✉) • A. Desai
Department of Neurosurgery, Stanford University, Stanford, CA, USA
e-mail: zmedress@stanford.edu; trinxile@stanford.edu; jratliff@stanford.edu; atman@stanford.edu

G. Tender (ed.), *Minimally Invasive Spine Surgery Techniques*,
https://doi.org/10.1007/978-3-319-71943-6_5

Contraindications

Patients who present with back pain or mechanical instability are unlikely to derive benefit from a minimally invasive laminectomy. Preoperative imaging that demonstrates deformity or high grade spondylolisthesis is a contraindication. Some surgeons believe that minimally invasive laminectomy may be performed in patients with non-mobile grade I spondylolisthesis without causing worsening instability. However, MIS laminectomy should be avoided in mobile or high grade spondylolisthesis as it may worsen instability. Prior surgery at the same level is a relative contraindication to an MIS approach given the presence of scar tissue and unpredictable tissue plans that may be difficult to navigate through a small operative corridor, though not an absolute contraindication.

Surgical Technique

The patient is positioned prone on a Wilson frame. All bony prominences should be adequately padded, and the abdomen should be allowed to hang freely in order to reduce venous hypertension and resultant epidural bleeding. The Wilson frame should be optimally positioned in order to increase intralaminar space. Using fluoroscopy, the appropriate level is identified and a skin incision is made 1–2 cm off midline. Bovie electrocautery is used to dissect to the level of the lumbodorsal fascia, which is sharply incised. The dilator is docked on the inferior lamina in a sweeping fashion in order to dissect away soft tissue. Lateral fluoroscopy is again used to confirm correct docking position on the inferior lamina of the superjacent level, and sequential dilators are used to sweep away soft tissue and introduce the tubular working channel. Soft tissue is remove from the lamina using bovie electrocautery and pituitary rongeurs. The laminectomy is performed with a high speed drill and kerrison rongeurs starting at the inferior lamina. The ligamentum flavum is dissected, undercut, and removed using a nerve hook, angled curettes, and kerrison rongeurs. The dura should be visibly decompressed, and meticulous hemostasis should be obtained in the epidural gutter using Floseal (Baxter, Deerfield, IL), Gelfoam (Pfizer, New York, NY), and cottonoids. Once adequate decompression has been obtained, the tubular retractor is slowly removed, and hemostasis is obtained using bipolar cautery in the muscular and subcutaneous layers through the tubular retractor given that areas of bleeding may be difficult to find after the retractor has been removed.

Of note, bilateral decompression can be accomplished from one side, docking only from one side and extending the bony removal to the deep part of the spinous process and contralateral lamina, achieving bilateral access in that fashion. Anterior-posterior fluoroscopy can be utilized when needed to confirm laterality (Figs. 5.1 and 5.2).

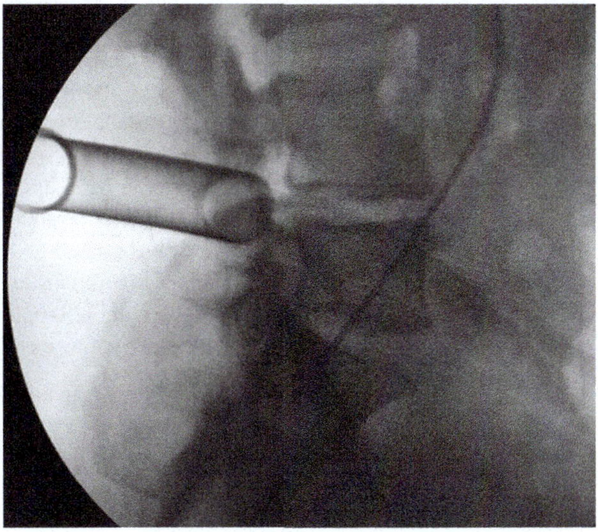

Fig. 5.1 Example docking for a L4–5 decompression

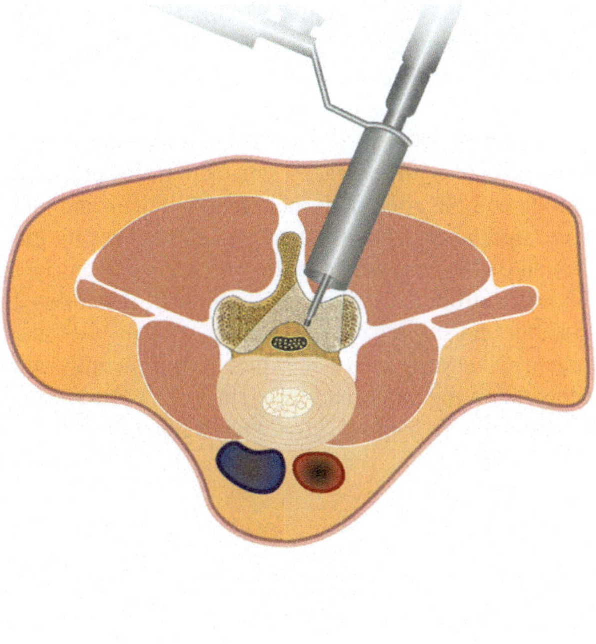

Fig. 5.2 Example approach to bilat decompression, MIS

Pearls and Pitfalls

Downward pressure should be maintained on the dilators at all time during docking to avoid unintentional migration of the working channel. Ideally, the inferior edge of the lamina should be centered in the operative field in order to serve as a anatomic landmark prior to drilling.

Complications

Potential complications from MIS laminectomy include wrong level surgery, durotomy, CSF leak, inadequate decompression, hematoma, nerve root injury, wound infection, creation of mechanical instability from overly aggressive bony removal. In cases where a durotomy has occurred, a MIS approach provides the benefit of involving less dead space and tissue disruption. In such cases, a primary dural repair may be achieved and a dural sealant may be used to reinforce a primary repair. In cases of durotomy, a water-tight fascial closure is mandatory, and may be aided by the use of a hyper-curved needle such as UR-6 (Ethicon, Sommerville, NJ). Conversion to open may be necessary in some cases if significant CSF leak is encountered.

Literature Review

Minimally invasive laminectomy remains a bread and butter procedure for the treatment of lumbar spinal stenosis. In the 1970s, Caspar and Yasargil introduced microsurgical techniques to the treatment of lumbar disc herniation [2]. In experienced hands, durotomy occurs in less than 5% of cases using a minimally invasive approach, and nearly 90% of patients are discharged within 24 h of the operation [3]. Meta-analysis of open versus MIS laminectomy demonstrate that MIS laminectomy is associated with increased satisfaction, lower blood loss, lower pain scores, and similar complication rates including CSF leak and infection, though MIS operations were significantly longer than open approaches by 11 min [4]. Bilateral decompression through a unilateral tubular MIS approach can be safely and efficiently achieved without introducing clinically significant instability [5]. Given the small working corridor and specialized instruments used in MIS laminectomy, there is a well-documented learning curve in which a significantly increased number of durotomy, reoperation rate, incorrect level surgeries occurred in the first 30 cases [6]. In addition, procedure length decreased as a function of the chronologic case number.

Conclusions

Minimally invasive laminectomy remains an effective technique in treating symptomatic central and lateral recess lumbar stenosis. As with open laminectomy, the ideal patient for this procedure presents with symptoms of neurogenic claudication or lumbar radiculopathy in the absence of back pain, mechanical instability, high-grade spondylolisthesis, or deformity. Benefits include a smaller skin incision, reduced muscle and midline tension band disruption compared to open approaches, earlier mobilization, and reduced hospital stay.

References

1. Weinstein JN, Lurie JD, Tosteson TD, Hanscom B, Tosteson AN, Blood EA, Birkmeyer NJ, Hilibrand AS, Herkowitz H, Cammisa FP, Albert TJ, Emery SE, Lenke LG, Abdu WA, Longley M, Errico TJ, Hu SS. Surgical versus nonsurgical treatment for lumbar degenerative spondylolisthesis. N Engl J Med. 2007;356(22):2257–70. https://doi.org/10.1056/NEJMoa070302.
2. Deutsche Gesellschaft für Neurochiurgie. In: Wüllenweber R, editor. Lumbar disc; adult hydrocephalus: proceedings of the 27th annual meeting of the Deutsche Gesellschaft für Neurochirurgie, Berlin, September 12–15, 1976, Advances in neurosurgery, vol. 4. Berlin: Springer; 1977.
3. Podichetty VK, Spears J, Isaacs RE, Booher J, Biscup RS. Complications associated with minimally invasive decompression for lumbar spinal stenosis. J Spinal Disord Tech. 2006;19(3):161–6. https://doi.org/10.1097/01.bsd.0000188663.46391.73.
4. Phan K, Mobbs RJ. Minimally invasive versus open laminectomy for lumbar stenosis: a systematic review and meta-analysis. Spine. 2016;41(2):E91–E100. https://doi.org/10.1097/brs.0000000000001161.
5. Palmer S, Turner R, Palmer R. Bilateral decompression of lumbar spinal stenosis involving a unilateral approach with microscope and tubular retractor system. J Neurosurg. 2002;97(2 Suppl):213–7.
6. Sclafani JA, Kim CW. Complications associated with the initial learning curve of minimally invasive spine surgery: a systematic review. Clin Orthop Relat Res. 2014;472(6):1711–7. https://doi.org/10.1007/s11999-014-3495-z.

Chapter 6
Minimally Invasive Transforaminal Lumbar Interbody Fusion

Daniel Serban, Niki Calina, Anthony Digiorgio, and Gabriel Tender

Introduction

Minimally invasive transforaminal lumbar interbody fusion (MI TLIF) is one of the most commonly performed minimally invasive spine operations in the United States. This technique involves an algorithm of operative steps that allows safe decompression and stabilization of the diseased segment.

Indications

The indications for MI TLIF are the same as for the open TLIF:

- Lumbar instability with grade 1 or 2 spondylolisthesis
- Discogenic pain, after failure of conservative treatment and adequate work-up
- At the bottom of a long construct, e.g., for deformity correction.

Electronic Supplementary Material The online version of this chapter https://doi.org/10.1007/978-3-319-71943-6_6. contains supplementary material, which is available to authorized users.

D. Serban • N. Calina
Department of Neurosurgery, "Bagdasar-Arseni" Hospital, Bucharest, Romania

A. Digiorgio
Department of Neurosurgery, Louisiana State University Health Sciences Center, New Orleans, LA, USA
e-mail: Adigi2@lsuhsc.edu

G. Tender (✉)
Louisiana State University, New Orleans, LA, USA

G. Tender (ed.), *Minimally Invasive Spine Surgery Techniques*,
https://doi.org/10.1007/978-3-319-71943-6_6

Common conservative treatments prior to considering surgical intervention include NSAIDs, physical therapy, epidural steroid injections etc. Diagnostic imaging typically starts with dynamic flexion-extension X-rays and MRI (or CT-myelogram, in patients who cannot have MRI). Further testing may include CT-SPECT [1], facet blocks, selective nerve root blocks, discogram etc.

In patients with apparent positive sagittal balance, scoliosis films and/or a full deformity work-up should be performed.

Contraindications

High-grade spondylolistheses (grade 3 or 4) should be treated by open, rather than MI, TLIF. In these cases, we often perform an open bilateral laminectomy and facetectomy, bilateral discectomy, reduction of the listhesis on the pedicle screws (inserted with bicortical purchase), and insertion of PLIF, rather than TLIF, cages.

A relative contraindication is morbid obesity, when the distance between the skin surface and the lamina is over 100 mm (the longest typical tubular retractor). However, since the fat is depressible, we have used this technique in many morbidly obese patients without having to convert to an open procedure.

Surgical Technique

The following operative steps are described:

- patient positioning
- skin incision
- graft harvesting
- retractor placement
- medial facetectomy
- lateral facetectomy and yellow ligament removal
- discectomy
- cage insertion
- ipsilateral pedicle screw insertion
- contralateral percutaneous pedicle screw insertion
- closure

Patient Positioning

The patient is placed in prone position with the arms tucked to the sides and with adequate padding for all pressure points. We take an AP image and adjust the table, not the C-arm, until the spinous process at the level of interest is perfectly centered between the two pedicles. We place the patient in slight reverse Trendelenburg position when we operate on the L5–S1 level, in order to have less of a cranio-caudal work angle. We do NOT flex the table, since the patient would be fused with a straight lumbar spine (instead of lordotic). In fact, we occasionally extend the lumbar spine (using the re-flex option of the surgical bed) *after* inserting the interbody cage, in order to restore some of the lumbar lordosis, in selected cases.

Skin Incision

The level of interest is identified on the lateral image by placing a spinal needle in alignment with the intervertebral disc of interest. The skin incision is centered on the spinal needle entry point, and is typically 2.5–3 cm in length, parallel to the midline and about 5–6 cm lateral to it. In patients with larger body habitus, the incision has to be placed further laterally. For the L5–S1 and the L4–5 levels, the most common levels treated, the skin incision is usually just above the iliac crest. After local hemostasis for the skin edges, the incision of the subcutaneous fat and the lumbar fascia is continued with the 10-blade in a lateral to medial direction, and maintaining the same cranial to caudal angulation as the localizing spinal needle, until the lumbar fascia is encountered.

Graft Harvesting

We prefer to use bone marrow aspirate (60 cc's, later to be concentrated to 7 cc's of mesenchymal cells, mixed with demineralized bone matrix to be used as fusion material) and occasionally autologous iliac crest graft (Video 6.1). The lumbar fascia inserts on the iliac crest; therefore, once we expose the fascia, we follow it caudally to its' insertion on the crest. Typically, the crest is found just caudal to the edge of the skin incision. We follow it medially until the posterior superior iliac spine (PSIS) is palpated. Then, a Jamshidi needle is inserted in the PSIS in a cranial to caudal and medial to lateral direction, in order to not violate the SI joint, located caudal to the PSIS. Upon aspiration, the bone marrow should come into the syringe slowly; we turn the needle by 90° every 15 s and occasionally advance it by half a centimeter every minute in order to maximize aspiration of bone marrow rather than just venous blood.

If autologous iliac crest graft is desired (e.g., in smokers or patients with osteoporosis), we use to self-retaining retractors to expose the fascia over the PSIS. Then, using either a trephine or dedicated instruments (e.g., the crest harvester by Globus Medical), a cylinder of bone about 3 cm long is extracted, using the same entry point and direction as described for the Jamshidi needle. In order to minimize postoperative pain, care must be exercised to respect the direction of the iliac crest, so that only the cancellous bone is harvested (i.e., the internal and external cortices must not be violated). Also, we do not go deeper than 3 cm with the harvester, since penetrating the sciatic notch would place the sciatic nerve at risk. Occasionally, when a larger amount of graft is needed, we harvest a second cylinder of cancellous bone just lateral to the first one, but with a separate cortical entry on the cranial edge of the iliac crest (i.e., we do NOT use the same entry hole, since that would decrease the volume of graft harvested). Hemostasis is then achieved with bone wax and Gelfoam soaked in Marcaine (for postoperative pain control). The fascia can usually be closed with a "figure of 8" 0-Vicryl on a UR needle.

Retractor Placement

The lumbar fascia is incised in a longitudinal fashion, parallel to the skin incision and slightly medial to it. The paraspinal muscles are then dissected in a lateral to medial direction, either with the index finger or with one of the small dilators.

There is an antero-posterior fascial layer, between the multifidus and the erector spinae muscles, that inserts on the tip of the lateral facet. If this fascial layer is not penetrated, the dilator will slide on its' lateral aspect and the retractor will be positioned laterally, on the junction of the lateral facet with the transverse process. In this case, the retractor is pulled out and, through the same fascial opening, the muscle fibers are penetrated more medially. Of course, the antero-posterior fascial layer, between the multifidus and the erector spinae muscles, has to be forcefully penetrated with the smaller dilator, so that the tip of the dilator lands on the lamina of interest. Occasionally, this fascial layer opening has to be enlarged by sharp dissection (i.e., scissors or Bovie cautery).

After sequential dilation and placement of the tubular or 2-blade retractor, there is typically a small amount of muscle fibers left on the lamina; this can be removed with pituitary rongeurs and Bovie cautery. In patients with hypertrophic facets, it may seem that the lamina is very deep in the exposed field; in these cases, it helps to get multiple lateral X-rays, showing that we are still superficial to the spinal canal, and start the exposure laterally, with the Bovie cautery, until the junction between the medial facet and the lamina is identified.

The correct placement of the retractor, in line with the intervertebral disc of interest, is confirmed with lateral fluoroscopy and then the retractor is locked in place with a rigid arm. Once the retractor is locked in place and the remaining muscle is removed, the operative microscope is brought into the field and the following structures should be exposed in the operative field: caudally, the caudal edge of the lamina of interest; medially, the junction between the lamina and the spinous process; laterally, the lateral aspect of the lateral facet; and in the center of the exposure, the pars interarticularis, with its characteristic appearance of a "valley" between two "hills" (the above and below joints). We prefer to enter the caudal joint with the Bovie cautery, to confirm the anatomic location and also to facilitate the removal of the medial facet later on.

There are some slight variations depending on the type of retractor used. The tubular retractor has the advantage of being compact and keeping the muscle out of the way circumferentially. The pedicle-based retractor is described in detail below (Video 6.3). The two-blade (cranio-caudal) retractor, with the option of adding a third, medial, blade, is the one we currently use most frequently, because it is simple, it allows towing of the blades for further cranio-caudal exposure (without enlarging the skin incision), and it allows for medial-lateral angulation of the curettes and rasps to prepare both the contralateral and ipsilateral endplates without adjusting the retractor (as is the case with the tubular retractor) (Video 6.4).

Medial Facetectomy

This step begins with two osteotomies: one vertical, parallel to the spinous process and just lateral to it, and the other one horizontal, through the pars interarticularis. We use the high-speed drill to perform all osteotomies, but some surgeons may prefer to use osteotomes. We prefer to start with the vertical osteotomy, since it is similar to the one performed for microdiscectomies and quite familiar to most surgeons. This is a relatively safe step, since the underlying yellow ligament protects the dura mater. The osteotomy is started at the caudal edge of the lamina and extended cranially until the end of the yellow ligament is encountered. This typically corresponds to the caudal aspect of the cranial pedicle on lateral X-ray and marks the point where the horizontal osteotomy should be started. The vertical osteotomy is usually performed close to the spinous process, in which case the lamina is thin and the yellow ligament is encountered after only a few mm of drilling (with the typical lamina-drilling sequence of cortical bone, cancellous bone, cortical bone, yellow ligament). This allows for good central and even contralateral decompression of the spinal canal (Video 6.2). If central decompression is not necessary, the vertical osteotomy can be performed further laterally, in order to minimize the amount of dura mater exposed. In this case, the lamina is thicker and the yellow ligament is encountered deeper and at a tangential angle, as it curves towards the lateral recess.

The horizontal osteotomy is typically started at the cranial end of the vertical osteotomy, where the end of the yellow ligament is observed. The osteotomy starts in the lamina and continues through the pars interarticularis, which is much thicker than the lamina. We recommend getting a lateral fluoroscopic image at this point, to make sure that the osteotomy is below the caudal edge of the cranial pedicle. Once the horizontal osteotomy is completed, the medial facet becomes loose (when the horizontal osteotomy completes the pars transection, it also gives a tactile "pop"). We detach the capsular ligaments with the Bovie cautery, which allows the medial facet to be removed en-bloc with large pituitary rongeurs. If the facet is too bulky, we sometimes transect it in two pieces with the high-speed drill, which makes it easier to remove. At this time, the shiny medial aspect of the lateral facet is exposed.

Lateral Facetectomy and Yellow Ligament Removal

We prefer to perform this step before removing the yellow ligament, in order to protect the dura mater during drilling. The tip of the lateral facet is removed with the high-speed drill from cranial to caudal. We take a lateral fluoroscopic image to determine the projection of the cranial edge of the caudal pedicle and we mark that on the shiny medial aspect of the lateral facet, since that represents the caudal extent of the lateral facet removal. The lateral extent of the facet removal is represented by the soft tissues, where the tortuous lumbar artery is invariably encountered; fortunately, bleeding from this artery can be easily controlled with the bipolar cautery.

Once the partial lateral facetectomy is complete, the bony work is done and we can proceed with the yellow ligament removal. A small up-biting curette is flipped under the yellow ligament and followed with a Kerrison rongeur to remove the ligament in a piece-meal fashion. At this point, the lateral edge of the dural sac and the takeoff of the spinal nerve are exposed. The epidural veins are often prominent and should be coagulated with the bipolar cautery and sharply transected. The safest point to start coagulating the epidural veins is just lateral to the take-off of the traversing spinal nerve.

Discectomy

A typical degenerated disc is about 8–12 mm in height. In these cases, we start the annulotomy just lateral to the dural sac and extend it laterally for about 10–15 mm, unless the exiting spinal nerve is in the way (as is the case in patients with spondylolisthesis). A disc herniation can be removed at this time, if present, as described in the previous chapter. Once the annulus is opened with the 11 blade, we prefer inserting a small smooth shaver, e.g. 8 mm, as deep as the contralateral annulus permits; this is a tactile feel, but we also confirm it with lateral fluoroscopy, as there is a tendency to stop too soon and thus not remove enough disc material. The shaver is rotated in the disc space both contra- and ipsi-laterally, in order to dislodge as much nucleus pulposus as possible, to be then removed with pituitary rongeurs. We then use smooth shavers of increasing size, until the proper fit is achieved (again, this is determined both by tactile feel and fluoroscopic guidance). It is of paramount importance to assess the adequate desired height of the anterior, rather than posterior, disc space, since the cage will need to be inserted anteriorly and thus provide a lordotic construct. The smooth shavers of increasing size can be used to open up the disc space, since they will not violate the endplates. Once most of the nucleus pulposus is removed, we proceed with the endplate preparation. We occasionally start with undersized sharp shavers, but most of the endplate preparation is done with wide rasps, so that we don't create troughs that would decrease mechanical resistance and promote subsidence. If the disc has significant lordosis (e.g., at L5–S1), it may seem difficult to insert a large cage (as dictated by the high anterior disc space) through the small posterior disc opening. In this case, we recommend using a sharp shaver with the same height as the anterior disc space and rotate it against the cage entry point in the posterior disc space; this, of course, requires protection of the lateral spinal sac, but if the annulotomy was started lateral to the spinal sac, usually no dural retraction is necessary. Alternatively, we can use expandable cages. Once the contra- and ipsi-lateral cranial and caudal endplates are prepared, copious irrigation with antibiotic solution is performed, prior to graft and cage insertion.

Cage Insertion

This is perceived as the most difficult step of the case, especially since we recommend inserting a cage approximately 2 mm taller than the anterior disc height. However, if the entry point for the cage is widened by using a sharp shaver of the same size as the anterior disc height, cage insertion becomes safe and easy.

Prior to cage insertion, we pack a large amount of graft material under pressure, in order to maximize the likelihood of fusion according to Wolff's law. In the mix, we use bone marrow aspirate concentrate, demineralized bone matrix, stem cells, and morselized local bone (i.e., medial facet). If bone substitutes were not available, we have used autologous cancellous bone, harvested as described above. Our protocol involves insertion of graft material until it completely fills up the empty space created by the discectomy. We then use a smaller trial (e.g., an 8 mm height trial when a 12 mm height cage will be inserted) to pack the graft and create space for the cage (which will further compact the graft). We occasionally use a larger trial (e.g., 11 mm height trial when a 12 mm height cage will be inserted) to make sure the cage will follow easily. The cage is then filled with graft material and inserted in the intervertebral space. We recommend getting the tip of the cage into the disc space with the cage inserter almost vertical; this way, the risk of the cage slipping between the posterior longitudinal ligament and the spinal sac is minimized. Once the tip of the cage is engaged into the disc space, we then drop the hand laterally, holding the inserter in a lateral to medial fashion, so that the cage crosses the midline inside the disc space.

Regarding cage insertion, several characteristics are important.

- Height. The cage should have a height 2–3 mm larger than the anterior disc height and should be inserted as far anteriorly as allowed by the anterior longitudinal ligament; this provides indirect decompression of the opposite side, decompresses the foramina, and allows for restoration of lordosis, if necessary.
- Position. We try to insert the cage across the midline, for the same reasons mentioned above (although we consider a cage that is slightly off to one side of the midline to be acceptable).
- Length. If additional lordosis is desired, we use a smaller length cage and we compress on the screws (before locking the caps on the rods). Otherwise, we use a lordotic cage that will fit the length of the disc space, without protruding posteriorly.

- Footprint. We currently use straight lordotic cages, but there are many options available. Obviously, the larger the footprint, the better the likelihood of a fusion and the smaller the risk of subsidence.
- Material. We currently use PEEK cages, but, again, Titanium-coated PEEK cages porous Titanium cages, and other combinations, are available and show promise.
- Dynamic (expandable) cages. The advantage of expandable cages is obvious—ease of insertion and, once placed anteriorly, ease of lordosis restoration. The downside is that, once the cage is expanded, the graft material may become loose and, according to Wolff's law, fusion rates may decrease. Therefore, in these cases, we recommend inserting more graft, preferably through the cage, after expansion (aka "backfill" of the cage).

After cage insertion, hemostasis is achieved with Gelfoam and/or Surgiflo. If a small cage was used, we occasionally insert more graft behind the cage, but with care not to have large bone chips potentially backing up against the spinal sac or nerve root.

At the end of the case, before fascia and skin closure, we always check one more time to make sure the bottom of the cage is well below the dural sac and the hemostasis is pristine.

Ipsilateral Pedicle Screw Insertion

We perform this step under direct visualization. First, the lateral to medial angle of the tubular or 2-blade retractor is decreased, since the direction of the pedicles is closer to vertical than the direction of cage insertion. We typically start with the caudal pedicle, since it is easier to cannulate. The entry point for the caudal pedicle screw is identified a couple of mm caudal to the corner created by the drilled edge of the lateral facet, the lateral aspect of the lateral facet, and the shiny medial aspect of the lateral facet. This entry point can also be slightly adjusted in the cranio-caudal direction based on the lateral fluoroscopic image. The cortex is broken with the tip of the high-speed drill and then a pedicle finder is used to cannulate the pedicle in a slight cranial to caudal and lateral to medial direction (each pedicle has slightly different anatomic angles, and we recommend evaluating the direction of the pedicle finder both under the microscope and from a macroscopic standpoint). The cranio-caudal direction is dictated by the lateral fluoroscopic image, whereas the lateral to medial angulation is dictated by the visualization of the lateral aspect of the spinal sac, as well as the general knowledge of pedicular direction and anatomy. When in doubt, an AP fluoroscopic image can be obtained when the tip of the pedicle finder reaches the bottom of the pedicle on the lateral fluoroscopic image, to confirm that the tip of the pedicle finder is still within the ring of the pedicle on the AP image, but this is rarely necessary. Once the tip of the pedicle finder passes the bottom of the pedicle on the lateral image, neuromonitoring is employed to confirm that stimulation of the pedicle finder at 10 mA yields no response (i.e., there is no medial wall breach). Once the path is created, the pedicle finder is removed and a K-wire is inserted in its place.

The cranial pedicle is slightly harder to cannulate. Sometimes, the tubular or 2-blade retractor has to be angled cranially to expose the entry point for the cranial pedicle. There is a tendency to start the pedicle cannulation too medial, since the exiting nerve is often visualized and the surgeon knows that the pedicle is right above that nerve. We used this technique initially (Video 6.5), but we currently advise against it, because it is difficult to estimate the thickness of the pedicle, especially under microscope. Instead, we recommend further exposure cranially and laterally, until the junction between the cranial transverse process and its corresponding lateral facet is identified. The transverse process base should be clearly identified with a Penfield, including its' cranial and caudal edge. Then, and only then, the entry point for the cranial pedicle screw can be created with the high-speed drill at the above-mentioned junction (slightly riding on the lateral facet). Similar to the caudal pedicle, this entry point can also be slightly adjusted in the cranio-caudal direction based on the lateral fluoroscopic image. The pedicle is then cannulated with the pedicle finder as described above for the caudal pedicle, and another K-wire is inserted at this level.

Once the K-wires are in place, we remove the tubular or two-blade retractor and the rest of the procedure is performed in a similar fashion to the percutaneous technique.

Contralateral Percutaneous Pedicle Screw Insertion

The accurate placement of the percutaneous pedicle screws is dependent of the quality of the radiologic images. Therefore, obtaining true AP and lateral images prior to skin incision is of utmost importance.

The AP image should be obtained first. The C-arm is locked at 90°, perfectly centered on the vertebral body of interest. This is particularly important if the patient has significant deformity, in which case the C-arm should be readjusted for each vertebral body. The spinous process of the vertebral body of interest should be centered between the two pedicle rings; otherwise, the table (NOT the C-arm) should be tilted left or right until the desired position is achieved. Then, the table is placed in reverse Trendelenburg until the superior endplate of the vertebral body of interest becomes a single line (this may not be feasible for S1 if the sacral slope is steep).

The lateral image is obtained next. If the AP image was perfect, now the posterior margin of the targeted vertebral body should appear as a single line. The perfect lateral image is obtained by "wagging" the C-arm until the two pedicles of the vertebral body of interest overlap. At this point, the superior and inferior endplates should also appear as a single line.

After this, the bony landmarks can be marked on patient's skin under AP fluoroscopy: the midline, the left and right pedicle lines, and the interpedicular line for the vertebral body of interest. The skin incision mirrors the opposite one and should be about 2.5 cm in length, vertical and centered on the interpedicular line, about 4–6 cm off the midline. This point is typically just lateral to the tip of the transverse process on the AP image. In large patients, the skin incision has to be made further lateral, in order to maintain the same lateral-to-medial angle of insertion.

The lumbar fascia is then incised with the knife or Bovie medial to the skin incision. It is important to remember that the fascia is the layer that limits the exploration of the deep bony landmarks. Continuing in the same lateral to medial direction, the index finger can be inserted to find the junction between the transverse process and the lateral facet. Typically, the lateral facet is first encountered (since it is the most superficial), and then the finger is allowed to slide lateral to it and land on the posterior aspect of the transverse process. If the incision is too small to accommodate a finger, the same landmarks can be identified with the tip of a Jamshidi needle, with the aid of frequent fluoroscopic images. The ideal docking point is at the junction of the transverse process with the lateral facet, as medial as allowed by the lateral facet. On the AP image, this point will appear just outside the pedicle ring; if it appears inside the pedicle ring, it is likely that the tip of the needle is actually riding high on the lateral facet, not on the transverse process. On the lateral image, the tip of the needle should be just above the ring of the transverse process, not high on the lateral facet, and the trajectory should pass through the pedicle, parallel to the endplates. If fine adjustments are necessary, the tip of the Jamshidi needle can be moved with both hands (for maximal control) in millimeter increments, on the base of the transverse process, until the desired position is achieved.

Once the correct docking point is obtained, the needle is gently tapped through the pedicle. For the lower lumbar pedicles, the direction is typically lateral to medial and cranial to caudal, but the angles vary with each level (see below). As the needle is advanced through the pedicle, there should be no increased resistance (that would signify cortical bone and therefore imminent pedicle wall breach). The most important images are obtained when the tip of the needle reaches the base of the pedicle on the lateral image; at this time, the tip of the needle should be still within the pedicle ring on the AP image.

At this time, neuromonitoring is usually employed. The shaft of the needle is stimulated, and a response of 10 mA or above signifies that the medial or inferior pedicle walls have not been breached.

A particular situation is encountered if the tip of the needle is very close to the medial border of the pedicle ring on the AP image, and neuromonitoring yields low responses (e.g., 4–7 mA). In this situation, it is likely that the needle has violated the lateral recess, which sometimes loops under the line of the pedicle ring. Therefore, it is recommended that the tip of the needle should be well within the pedicle ring on the AP images, when it reaches the base of the pedicle on the lateral images.

Another important technical tool is changing the direction of the Jamshidi needle while in the pedicle. Indeed, if the original trajectory is angled too much lateral to medial, and the tip of the needle gets too close to the medial border of the pedicle on the AP image, the angulation of the needle can be changed to a more straight trajectory, without withdrawing the needle from the pedicle. The angulation can also be changed in a cranio-caudal direction, in order to keep the needle parallel to the endplates. Beveled needles are particularly useful in this situation, since they naturally change direction depending on the bevel orientation.

Once the needle trajectory is deemed safe, the tip of the needle is advanced into the vertebral body for a couple of centimeters, and then the center part of the needle is removed and a K-wire is inserted for about another centimeter past the tip of the Jamshidi needle, in order to stabilize it to the cancellous bone and make it less likely to inadvertently come out during the placement of the tap and screw. Then, the Jamshidi needle is removed, while the K-wire is kept in place with the other hand.

After this, most systems have a series of tubular dilators that slide over the K-wire; the outer dilator and the K-wire are kept in place, whereas the inner dilators are removed to make room for the tap and screw. The tap is then advanced over the K-wire into the pedicle of the vertebral body; it is sufficient (and recommended) to tap only past the base of the pedicle and not all the way into the vertebral body. For biomechanical reasons, we recommend undertapping by 2 mm (i.e., use a 4.5 mm tap for a 6.5 mm screw), in order to maintain the good purchase of the screw into the bone. It is important to maintain the direction of the K-wire with the tap; if the tap is not aligned with the K-wire, the part of the K-wire in the vertebral body starts to bend at the tip of the tap, and when a critical angle is reached, the tap cannot advance any more, and any further turns of the tap do nothing but strip (and destroy) the pedicle.

The tap is then removed and the screw (typically 6.5 × 45 mm for the average person) is inserted over the K-wire. Some surgeons prefer to insert all the K-wires in their respective pedicles before inserting the screws. Once the tip of the screw passes the base of the pedicle, the K-wire can be removed, and the screw further inserted through the previously created trajectory. The screw insertion must stop just before the head of the screw abuts the lateral facet; otherwise, the screw head loses its' poliaxial capabilities and makes subsequent rod insertion more difficult. All the screws have extender blades attached to their heads, in order to facilitate rod placement.

The second pedicle is cannulated in a similar fashion. A useful trick, particularly at L5–S1, is to perform the dissection with the index finger by moving it from the entry point of L5 to the entry point of S1; this also creates a working plane over which the rod can be easily inserted.

S1 The S1 pedicle is the largest. The transverse process equivalent in the sacrum is the ala, so the docking point for this level is found at the junction between the sacral facet and the ala. On the routine AP image, the tip of the needle will appear cranial and lateral to the pedicle ring, and just outside of it. On the lateral image, it will appear somewhat caudal. Since the pedicle is so large, there are a couple of options in choosing the entry point. One option involves starting the pedicle cannulation close to its cranial aspect and keeping the trajectory parallel to the endplate; this is the usual placement of screws ipsilateral to an MI TLIF construct, where the entry point is already exposed. The other option involves starting the cannulation more caudally and aim towards the sacral promontorium; this option is used when the distance between the L5 and S1 screw heads needs to be wider (e.g., for performing an MI TLIF using the pedicle-based retractor technique). It also allows for insertion of longer screws with better bone purchase, since the sacral lip has extremely hard bone.

The S1 pedicle is typically cannulated at 30° in the lateral-medial direction and about 30–60° in the cranial to caudal direction (this angle varies with the sacral tilt).

L5 The L5 pedicle is probably the hardest to cannulate, due to its small size and often sclerotic bone, as well as the fact that the pedicle image is partially masked by the iliac crest on the lateral X-ray. The docking point is usually close to the S1 one, and we prefer to place the L5 pedicle screw as cranial in the pedicle as possible, not only to avoid damage to the L5 spinal nerve exiting around the infero-medial aspect of the pedicle, but also to offer more space between the L5 and S1 pedicle screw heads (e.g., for an MI TLIF using the pedicle-based retractor technique).

The L5 pedicle is typically cannulated at 25–30° in the lateral-medial direction and 10–20° in the cranial to caudal direction.

L4 The L4 pedicle is usually larger than L5 and easy to identify on the lateral image. The L4 pedicle is typically cannulated at about 15–20° in the lateral-medial direction and close to 0° ("straight down") in the cranial to caudal direction.

Once the pedicle screws are in place, the rod must be placed on top of the screw heads and locked in place. Rod insertion can be done in three different ways, depending on the system.

The first way involves inserting the rod through a separate stab wound (e.g., Sextant/Longitude of Medtronic). One of the advantages of these systems is that it preserves the fascia and soft tissues between the towers. Another advantage (Sextant) is that it provides the most precise spondylolisthesis reduction. Finally, the Longitude system may provide easier navigation of the rod through the multiple towers. The main disadvantage of Sextant is that 2-level fixation is difficult (and 3-level is almost impossible). Another disadvantage is the additional skin incisions made for rod insertion.

The second way involves inserting the rod through either the cranial or the caudal tower (e.g., Revolve of Globus, ES2 of Stryker, Viper of Depuy-Acromed, Serengeti of K2M). The advantage is that it does not need an additional skin incision. The disadvantage is that it is somewhat more difficult to pass through all the towers, particularly in multilevel cases.

The third way involves dropping the rod through the towers (e.g., Spherx DBR of Nuvasive). This can only be done for a maximum of 2-level fusions. The disadvantage is that the tissues between the towers have to be disrupted; however, these tissues are already violated during screw placement. The advantage is that the rod has no overhang, and therefore the adjacent joints (particularly the cranial one) are somewhat protected from further degeneration (at least theoretically).

Regardless of the insertion method, the rod is then locked to the screw heads with appropriate caps. Most current systems have built-in reduction capabilities, which preclude the need for persuaders and can be used to reduce deformity curves. Once the rod is locked in place, the towers are removed from the screw heads and the wounds are closed in layers.

Closure

After removal of the towers, final hemostasis of the muscle is performed with the bipolar cautery at high voltage, under microscopic visualization. We perform a final examination of the spinal sac and the bottom of the cage, and we place Gelfoam over the exposed dura mater. Exparel can be injected in the paraspinous muscles for postoperative pain control.

The would is closed in layers with interrupted 2-0 Vycril on a UR needle for the lumbar fascia, followed by 3-0 Vycril and running subcutaneous 4-0 Monocryl for the skin.

Pearls and Pitfalls

Learning the MI Technique After Extensive Experience with the Open Technique

Most surgeons are initially trained in the open TLIF technique. The main difference with the MI technique, besides the limited field of view, is the angle of approach: in the open approach, the surgeon looks straight down at the laminae, the spinal sac, and the disc, whereas in the MI technique, these structures are approached obliquely. This difference is particularly important at the time of cage insertion. In the open technique, an effort is made to turn the cage in order for it to cross the midline; in the MI technique, just following the direction of the tubular retractor will take the cage across the midline. A common mistake made by the "open" surgeons when attempting their first MIS cases is to try to angle the cage even further; this can lead to insertion of the cage between the posterior longitudinal ligament and the dural sac (especially if the annular opening is not wide enough and the tip of the cage catches the medial annulus) or just anterior to the posterior longitudinal ligament, which of course is a suboptimal position. This is the reason we recommend holding the cage inserter almost vertical until the tip of the cage engages into the annular opening, and then dropping the hand laterally to drive the cage anteriorly in a lateral to medial direction, across the midline.

Skin Incision and Angle of Approach

There is some variability among MIS surgeons in terms of their preference on how lateral to place the skin incision. Obviously, the further lateral the skin incision, the more oblique the angle of approach. This lateral incision makes it a bit more difficult to place the retractor on the lamina and the surgeon has to angle the microscope throughout the case, but the advantages are that the cage is inserted at a more oblique lateral to medial angle, thus requiring less (or no) dural exposure and retraction, and the pedicle screw insertion is also easier, as the position of the pedicles is more lateral. If the skin incision is placed more medial, it is easier to dock on the lamina, but the laminectomy has to be extended medially and the dural sac has to be retracted in order to insert the cage. We prefer to use this more medial incision in patients with spondylolisthesis, when dural retraction is mandatory to achieve sufficient exposure to insert the cage.

The Pedicle-Based Retractor Technique

This is a variation of the MI TLIF technique in which the pedicle screws are inserted first [2]. We prefer using 2 C-arms for the placement of the K-wires in the respective pedicles, similar to the setup for a kyphoplasty. This technique is particularly useful when performing a 2-level TLIF, since all 6 K-wires can be inserted at the beginning of the case. The pedicle screws on the side of the TLIF have retractor blades attached to them, rather than screw heads; these screws are left slightly proud when inserted, to allow some mobility of the blades (otherwise, if the screws are driven all the way down in the pedicle, the blades hit the lateral facet and become difficult to mobilize). The retractor blades are then lined up with the direction of the disc (based on lateral fluoroscopy) and then locked in place with a rigid arm. The microscope is brought into the operative field and the same elements are exposed, from lateral to medial, as in the tubular retractor technique: the lateral and medial facets, the pars interarticularis, and the lamina. A third retractor blade is typically used medially to hold back the multifidus muscle against the spinous process. The main difference with this retractor is that the angle of approach is more acute than with the tubular retractor; therefore, care must be exercised not to insert the cage too far onto the contralateral side. After the laminectomy, discectomy, and cage insertion, the retractor blades are detached from the screw posts, the screw heads are attached, and the rod with the appropriate caps is locked in place.

L5–S1

This is the most common level to be treated.

We place the patient in reverse Trendelenburg to decrease the angle of view throughout the case.

In patients with a steep sacral slope, the skin incision must be made very high, in order to remain in line with the direction of the disc. In these patients, an effort must be made to insert the shavers against the S1 endplate, as the tendency is for the shavers to hit and damage the L5 endplate.

The L5 lamina is very wide and, if contralateral decompression is not needed, we prefer to place the vertical osteotomy more lateral, towards the medial facet, and only expose the lateral aspect of the dural sac after yellow ligament removal.

This level is particularly important because it provides most of the lumbar lordosis. Therefore, the cage height must be planned to match the anterior disc height, despite the fact that the smaller posterior disc height may make cage insertion difficult. Another option is to use expandable cages.

Additional lordosis can be used by gently compressing on the screws; however, excessive compression on the screws may lead to contralateral L5 nerve compression and radiculopathy, since the contralateral foramen has not been directly decompressed.

Sacral (S1) Posterior "Lip"

This is a common anatomical variation (or result of degeneration), in which a posterior S1 osteophyte ("lip") blocks the access to the disc space. In these cases, we recommend using the high-speed drill to remove the sacral lip starting at the lateral edge of the spinal sac and extending it laterally for about 1.5 cm or until the exiting spinal nerve is encountered. As the drilling continues in the depth, the soft disc material is encountered. This allows for insertion of the shavers and the discectomy is continued as described above.

L4–5

This level can usually be treated by both MI TLIF and LLIF. We prefer using the LLIF whenever possible. However, the MI TLIF must still be used when there is an associated large disc herniation or when the LLIF is not technically feasible.

The L4 lamina is narrower than L5, but typically still allows for a safe TLIF, without much dural sac retraction. However, the vertical osteotomy must be done medially, at the base of the spinous process.

While the L4–5 disc is typically not as lordotic as the L5–S1, an effort must be made at this level as well, to match the cage height to the anterior disc height.

L3–4 and L2–3

We recommend using the LLIF technique to fuse these levels whenever possible. The MI TLIF technique is dangerous at these levels because the lamina is very narrow and significant dural retraction is necessary in order to insert the cage. If MI TLIF must be used (e.g., retroperitoneal scarring), we recommend extensive bony removal, from the medial aspect of the lamina to the lateral aspect of the lateral facet, and spinal sac retraction to allow for insertion of an adequate size cage.

Spondylolisthesis

These cases are more difficult because the exiting spinal nerve often limits the space available for cage insertion laterally. Therefore, in these cases, we make room by retracting the spinal sac medially. This is done by performing a full hemilaminectomy, i.e., the vertical osteotomy is made at the base of the spinous process and the yellow ligament is removed over the entire half of the exposed spinal canal. Once the epidural veins are coagulated and transected, the dural sac is retracted medially with a nerve root retractor and increasing size smooth shavers are used to perform the discectomy.

It is important to angle the shavers towards the caudal endplate (e.g., the S1 endplate for the L5–S1 disc), otherwise the shaver may hit the back of the slipped cranial vertebral body (L5 in the example above). The same angulation towards the caudal endplate is maintained when inserting the trial and then the cage. This is a good indication for expandable cages, since the available space for insertion is limited and, particularly at L5–S1, a large lordotic cage must be placed in the anterior disc space.

Once the cage is in place, the spondylolisthesis is already partially reduced. The case is finished by using the percutaneous pedicle screw reduction system to complete the realignment.

Previous Discectomy

Patients who had a previous open discectomy and need a fusion at that level may benefit from the MI technique. In fact, because of the different angle of approach, the MI TLIF can be performed almost identically to a non-operated patient. The only part where the surgeon may encounter some scarring is at the time of the medial facetectomy, since the yellow ligament was probably removed at the time of the initial discectomy.

Collapsed Disc

When the disc is almost completely collapsed, or when there is a shell of calcification or cortical bone covering the annulus, it may seem difficult to access the disc. In these cases, we use the high-speed drill to remove a thin layer of bone along with the osteophytes (if present) starting at the lateral edge of the spinal sac and progressing laterally for about 1.5 cm. This allows for exposure of the posterior-most aspect of the two hard surfaces of the cranial and caudal endplates. We prefer to insert the smallest smooth shaver (5 mm height, if available) both in the contralateral disc space as well as the ipsilateral one. If the disc space does not open to make room for small shaver, we have used an osteotome instead, just to allow for the subsequent insertion of the shavers. We then use smooth shavers of increasing size, to open up the disc space without violating the endplates. It is important to insert the shavers as deep as possible, without violating the opposite annulus of course, in order to have increased leverage when opening up the disc space by turning the shavers. Often times, a 10 mm height cage is sufficient in these cases, since their starting disc height is less than 5 mm.

Normal Height Disc

These are typically patients with pars defects and grade 1 or 2 spondylolisthesis, but with preserved disc height and often with large disc herniations.

Obviously, the higher the disc, the more difficult it is for the graft to turn into bridging bone between the two endplates. We compensate in these cases by preparing a large fusion surface (both on the contra- and ipsi-lateral sides) and of course by thoroughly preparing the endplate surfaces. It is not uncommon to pack 10–15 cc's of graft before inserting the cage in these cases. Finally, the cage needed is often 15 or 16 mm in height.

Two-Level MI TLIF

Most commonly, this is done at L4–5 and L5–S1. The advantage is that both levels can be done through the same skin incision, since only the angle of the retractor changes from one level to the other.

If the *tubular retractor* is used, we prefer to start with the L5–S1 level. Once the cage is inserted, we recommend cannulating the S1 pedicle as described above and leaving a K-wire in. The retractor tube is then removed and reinserted to expose the level above (L4–5), leaving the S1 K-wire outside the retractor. The L4–5 TLIF is then performed and the L5 and L4 pedicles are cannulated as described above. K-wires are placed in these pedicles as well, and the retractor is removed and the procedure is completed in a percutaneous fashion.

If the *pedicle-based retractor* is used, the retractor blades are placed on the cranial and caudal screw posts (on the L4 and S1 screw posts in the example above). The L5 screw post is also inserted in the L5 pedicle, but without the head, since that would interfere with the exposure and cage insertion. The TLIFs are then performed through the same retractor, by adequately changing the direction of the retractor for L5–S1 and then L4–5. The screw heads, the rod, and the caps, are all placed at the end of the procedure, after the TLIFs are done.

Unilateral Pedicle Screws

The literature suggests that unilateral fixation after TLIF is not biomechanically as strong as the bilateral fixation, but the clinical results are similar. We occasionally recommend MI TLIF with unilateral, ipsilateral, pedicle screw fixation, in young patients who have good quality bone, have a large amount of osteoprogenitor cells in their bone marrow, and are likely to fuse in record time. In these cases, we often insert long screws with bicortical purchase.

Direction of the Pedicle Screw Heads

Regardless of the technique used, just before the final tightening of the caps on the screw heads, we recommend bringing the screw heads as close to the midline as possible, so that they can be easier to access, in case an open approach is needed in the future (e.g., to extend the fusion cranially or caudally).

Postero-Lateral (Intertransverse) Grafting

We only perform postero-lateral grafting in patients at high risk for non-union (e.g., smokers). The ipsilateral grafting is easy, since the base of the transverse process or ala are already exposed and slight angulation of the retractor laterally allows for exposure of the entire length of the transverse process or ala, followed by decortication and graft placement.

The contralateral side can only be grafted if the minimally invasive retractor is used to expose the transverse processes (or sacral ala). In these cases, the screws can be inserted similarly to the ipsilateral side, with the entry points started with the high-speed drill under direct visualization.

Complications

Dural Tear

Inadvertent durotomies can occur, particularly in difficult cases (spondylolisthesis, extreme degeneration etc). Due to the limited exposure, a direct repair with 4-0 Nurolon is rarely feasible. We prefer to temporarily cover the durotomy with a Gelfoam and patty, and complete the TLIF. At the end, we place a small piece of DuraGuard or DuraMatrix over the durotomy and then cover with DuraSeal. Most often, due to the sealing effect of the muscle, a CSF fistula is not observed. In the few cases in which a CSF fistula does occur, we prefer placing a lumbar drain for 5–7 days, rather than re-exploring the wound.

Nerve Injury

The nerve structure most frequently injured, particularly if spondylolisthesis is present, is the exiting spinal nerve (e.g., the L4 nerve when performing an L4–5 MI TLIF). The reason is that this nerve is relatively fixed against the corresponding pedicle and therefore cannot be retracted out of the way. The only way to protect this nerve is to limit the annulotomy just medial to the exiting spinal nerve and extend it medially under the spinal sac, if needed to insert a larger cage. In patients with grade 2 spondylolisthesis, this maneuver still allows for insertion of an appropriate size cage, whereas in grade 3 or 4, there is not enough space, hence the relative contraindication.

Another possible nerve injury can be caused by excessive compression on the screw heads. The injury typically occurs on the contralateral side, where the nerve was not directly decompressed by facetectomy.

Finally, the exposed dura mater can be compressed by a postoperative hematoma (particularly if a dural tear occurred, allowing for the CSF pressure to decrease and potentially allow the epidural veins to bleed in the postoperative period). If the dura was extensively exposed (e.g., in patients with spondylolisthesis or if contralateral decompression was necessary) and a postoperative compressive hematoma occurs, a cauda equina syndrome can ensue. That is the main reason we recommend limiting the dural exposure to the minimum necessary. In most cases, only a small area of the lateral spinal sac needs to be exposed, so even if a postoperative hematoma occurs, only minimal or no deficits would ensue.

Misplacement of Ipsilateral Pedicle Screws

This is rare and usually occurs at the cranial pedicle, due to an entry point that is too medial (i.e., the entry point is chosen on the drilled aspect of the former pars interarticularis rather than at the junction between the transverse process and lateral facet. Besides AP fluoroscopy, showing the medial position of the tip of the pedicle finder, neuromonitoring also signals the problem by yielding values of less than 10 mA. If only the Jamshidi needle was inserted, the solution is simple – a new entry point is chosen at the correct location and a new, proper trajectory is created. However, if the pedicle screw was inserted in the incorrect position and the pedicle is small (e.g., L5), it may be impossible to create a second trajectory lateral to the original one. In these cases, a "cortical screw" trajectory can be attempted, starting medially at the junction between the pars interarticularis and the lateral facet and aiming "up and out", similar to the cervical lateral mass screws. This maneuver is difficult with tubular retractors and slightly easier with the two-blade retractor.

Massive Blood Loss

This is a rare and unfortunate complication that results from damage to the great abdominal vessels after penetration of the anterior annulus fibrosus by sharp or biting instruments. While we have not encountered this complication, it is recommended that, if vascular damage occurs, the patient should be turned immediately in supine position and abdominal exploration, preferably by a general or vascular surgeon, should be performed in order to stop the bleeding.

Construct Failure

This complication refers to migration of the screws into their respective pedicles and occasionally re-slippage after a reduced spondylolisthesis. The treatment has to be individualized depending on the characteristics of each case, but typically involve additional levels of fixation.

Cage Retropulsion

This complication is rare and involves delayed migration of a cage posteriorly. If the cage was inserted without any dural retraction, its' posterior migration may remain asymptomatic, as no neural structures are stretched. However, if the bottom of the cage elevates or medially displaces the traversing spinal nerve (e.g., the S1 nerve for an L5–S1 TLIF), the patient will experience radiculopathy in that distribution. In these cases, we recommend re-exploring and removing the cage through the same incision, followed by an alternative way to insert an interbody graft (e.g., ALIF for L5–S1 or LLIF for L4–5) (Fig. 6.1).

Pseudarthrosis

With proper technique, less than 10% of the MI TLIF patients should experience pseudarthrosis. Symptomatic patients can be revised by either an alternative way to insert an interbody graft (e.g., ALIF for L5–S1 or LLIF for L4–5) or by the addition of a postero-lateral, intertransverse, fusion (in which case we typically use rhBMP).

Adjacent Level Disease

This is a delayed complication that typically occurs at least 5–10 years after the original fusion. Before addressing the respective level with a fusion, we recommend obtaining standing scoliosis films, to confirm that the adjacent level failure is not related to positive sagittal balance.

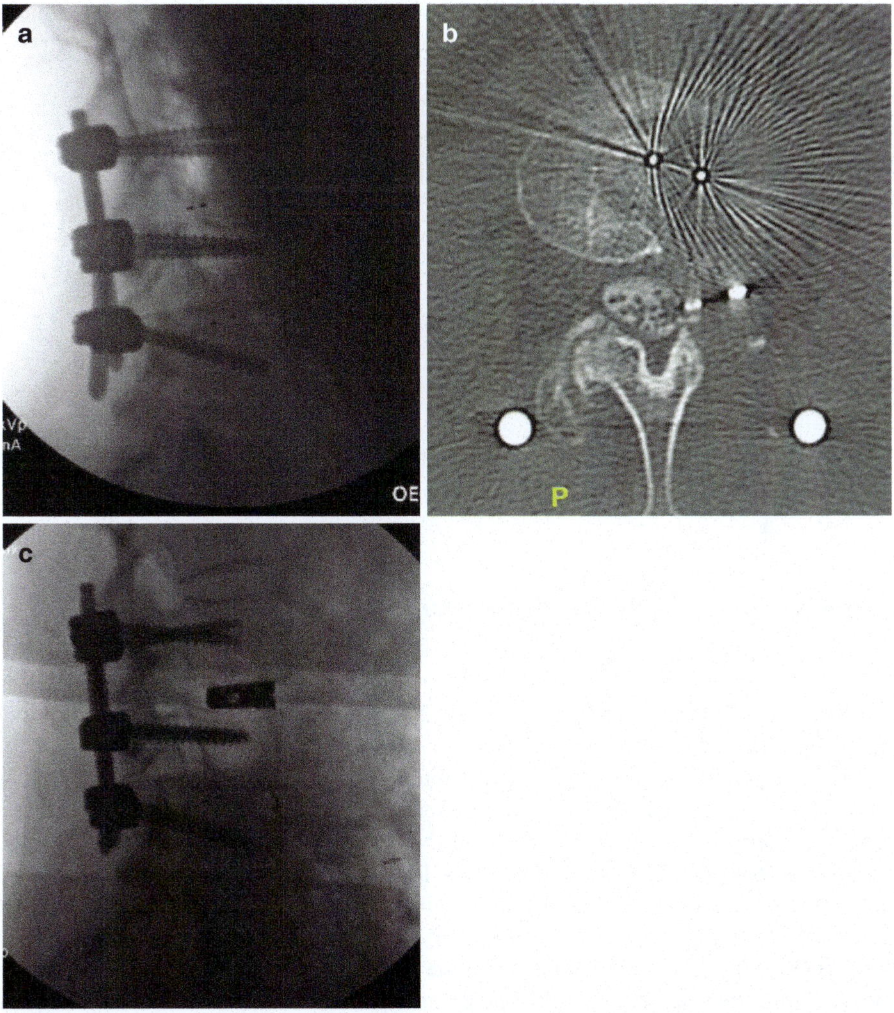

Fig. 6.1 Cage retropulsion at L3–4 after MI TLIF at L3–4, 4–5. (**a**) Intraoperative imaging showing adequate placement of the instrumentation. (**b**) Imaging at 3 months postoperatively showing retropulsion of the L3–4 cage. (**c**) Intraoperative imaging showing removal of the L3–4 cage (through the same incision) and placement of an MIS lateral expandable cage

Literature Review

There are many retrospective studies comparing MI versus open TLIF, with most of them showing MI TLIF advantages, including: decreased blood loss, decreased infection rate, decreased postoperative pain medication usage, lower cost, and shorter hospital stay [3–10]. These retrospective studies are prone to selection and recall bias, however.

Wang et al. [11] published the results of a prospective randomized study and concluded that the patients in the MI group experienced less sacrospinalis muscle injury, resulting in early functional recovery and superior short-term treatment effects. However, they found similar long-term efficacy for the two groups.

We published some of our results in a prospective randomized study [12]. The only significant benefit we found was the shorter hospital stay. This likely explains the cost savings found in previous studies, as reduction in stay by just one day can save upwards of $3000 in an American hospital.

Nonetheless, patients seem to favor the MI technique, when the two options are offered. In addition, as surgeons become more familiar with the minimally invasive techniques, operative time & blood loss decrease while outcomes improve [13].

Conclusions

When compared to the open TLIF, the MI TLIF technique offers similar clinical improvement and fusion rates, but with shorter hospital stay.

Addendum: Informative Letter to the Patients

The following informative letter is NOT intended to cover ALL the possible complications and scenarios. It is only intended to serve as a general guide, to improve patients' understanding of the operation.

This procedure can be very long. Despite careful padding of all pressure points, abrasions and pressure sores can occur. Generally these are minor, but can be serious, especially if they occur on the face. Nerve damage, particularly at the joints, can also occur. Blood clots forming in the legs, with potential death from spread to the lungs, are always a worry, and we use special inflatable devices to minimize that risk. Blood loss during this kind of surgery is normal and unavoidable, and sometimes we need to give transfusions from the blood bank. All of the blood is carefully tested, but unfortunately no test is perfect and there is always a small risk of acquiring some disease, such as hepatitis or AIDS. Death from anesthesia reaction or massive blood loss is possible, but fortunately extremely rare.

We make a one-inch skin incision in the lower back, usually on the side of the worse leg pain. Before we go to the spine, we use this incision to take a small amount of your pelvic bone with a special device that preserves the outer part of the bone and minimizes pain after surgery. Nevertheless, it is common to experience pain and soreness at the site where bone graft has been harvested. Sometimes this is permanent. Damage to small nerves in the area can lead to numbness or even pain over the buttocks.

We then reach the spinal column with a small tube, under x-ray guidance. At this point, an operating microscope is used to allow us to keep the incision as small as possible, yet have excellent vision so we can see what needs to be done. We remove some of the bone in the back of the spine (i.e., laminectomy and facetectomy) and then we remove the bad disc or discs and prepare the area to accept the fusion construct. If pinched nerves are present causing pain in the legs, then bone and disc material is removed as needed to take the pressure off of the nerves. When previous surgery has been done, scar tissue is always present. Sometimes this scar tissue can be very thick and tough, and getting through it to find the nerves increases the risk of nerve damage and spinal fluid leakage. After we take out the disc, we replace it with a synthetic box we call "cage" that is filled up with bone graft and will promote the bony fusion. We are careful to avoid damage to the nerves in the spinal canal, which are very close to our "working area". However, such damage (while very rare) is a risk and can result in paralysis from nerve damage, loss of bowel, bladder, and sexual function, numbness, lack of feeling or sensation, or even severe pain below the waist. X-rays are used throughout the procedure to maximize the safety.

In order to give instant strength and stability to the spine and to increase the probability of the natural bony fusion healing properly, we use metal screws and rods. We place the screws accurately with the aid of intraoperative x-ray guidance. Nerve or blood vessel damage is possible, but fortunately quite rare. These devices function as an internal cast to keep the spinal bones immobile while the bone cells are forming the fusion mass. (If you're gluing two pieces of wood together, the glue is more likely to stick if you keep the wood pieces in a vice until the glue is set.) The screws and rods have been engineered and designed for endurance, but if a natural bony fusion does not form, eventually they will work loose or break. Another risk of any type of implanted foreign (non-natural) body is the possibility of infection. If this occurs (which is rare) it is early, and not months or years later. Generally removal of the screws is not necessary (to treat the infection), but prolonged antibiotics and debriding (cleaning up) procedures could be required.

It is important that you understand that this is a serious and possibly painful operation with a long and slow recovery. Most frequently, after the surgery you will be moved from the recovery room to a normal hospital room. Occasionally, if the surgery takes longer than a few hours, you may need to be monitored in the intensive care unit. Sometimes the intestines are sluggish for a few days and until you begin to "pass gas", your intake of food may be restricted. We encourage you to walk with assistance as soon as possible, and it is hoped that the total hospital stay will be in the range of 1–4 days. Of course, this is varied as needed on an individual basis.

At home we would encourage a program of walking on a level surface, gradually increasing the distance to between 2 and 3 miles a day. At about 3 months, a home exercise regimen can be cautiously started. Return to daily activities is highly variable, but in general it is sometimes possible to return to the equivalent of a light office type job at about that time (3 months). Maximal medical improvement is generally reached around a year after the date of surgery. It is generally not advised to engage in heavy manual labor type occupations following an operation of this nature.

Over the 6–12 months after surgery, it is hoped that the operated discs will heal and grow into a strong bony mass, so as to cause a solid union between the bones. This is a gradual process and at first there is no increased strength. This healing process is dependent upon the patient's powers of healing and does not always occur properly. The use of nicotine in any form (cigarettes, smokeless tobacco, nicotine patches, or nicotine gum) interferes with bone healing and dramatically decreases the odds of a successful fusion. You should not smoke or use nicotine in any form! Generally about 3 months is required for the fusion to begin to set, but strengthening continues for about a year or more. Also, for the first several months after surgery it is best to avoid non-steroidal anti-inflammatory drugs (such as aspirin, Motrin, Aleve, Naprosyn, etc.). These medications may interfere with bone healing. Tylenol use is OK, but you should be careful not to exceed the recommended dose. We expect to achieve a successful fusion for one disc level in about 90% and for two levels in about 80%. Sometimes postoperative x-rays show that the fusion has not healed to form solid bone. Most of the time, this does not seem to matter because a tough scar tissue-like gristle has formed instead and there are no symptoms. Occasionally, however, the failed fusion is symptomatic. That is called a pseudoarthrosis and repeat surgery is sometimes required. The type of surgery in those cases depends on individual circumstances.

Major complications (life threatening) may occur in about 2% of cases. The most common major complication is implant malposition or migration and may require reoperation. Sudden massive blood loss could occur, resulting in death. Other major complications include pneumonia and pulmonary embolism (blood clot going to the lungs).

There is also the chance that another type of fusion operation will be required if this one does not heal solidly. For example, it might be necessary to perform an additional operation in the side or front of the spine, with more bone graft added at that time. In some patients, only 360° (front and back) fusions are sufficient to give adequate strength for their particular spinal problem.

One last potential problem after fusion surgery is what we call "juxtafusional disease". After you have had a successful spinal fusion, that segment becomes immobile and the joints above and/or below that fusion are subjected to increased stress. Over the years, these joints can have problems that may require further surgery.

It is very important to emphasize that no operation or device is a "spine transplant". Results on an individual basis cannot be predicted, and therefore we certainly cannot give any guarantees or promises. Once you have a bad back, you always will have a bad back to some degree. You could be no better, or even worse. Most patients indicate that *on average* the pain is improved from "marked" to "mild". While this is a great improvement, it is usually not improved to "occasional" or "none". Whether you will be able to return to their pre-injury or preoperative level of functioning will have to be determined on an individual basis. As a general rule, it is about a year before patients are "over" the operation because recovery and reconditioning is a slow process. It is sometimes necessary to call upon the Departments of Physical Medicine & Rehabilitation and Occupational Medicine to perform functional capacity evaluations (FCE) to determine a patient's actual limitations and abilities.

My general advice to anyone with a spinal affliction of this nature is to "live with it "(if possible). Of course that's easy for me to say because I'm not the one hurting. This operation has been recommended in the belief that your condition is serious and therefore taking the risks of surgery makes sense. I believe this is a good operation that is the best choice for your particular problem. If your only affliction is pain, the decision is yours and yours alone as to whether you can live with it. While I obviously hope and believe that this operation will help you, I cannot give any guarantees or promises about results. It is possible that you could be the same or even worse. Furthermore, my general recommendation is to "live with it" if possible and avoid the risks and uncertainties of surgery. Nevertheless I am offering my surgical services in an attempt to help you, but the decision to proceed is up to you.

References

1. Tender G, Constantinescu A, Conger A, DiGiorgio A. Primary pain generator identification by CT-SPECT in a patient with low back pain: a case report. BMC Res Notes. 2017;10:132. https://doi.org/10.1186/s13104-017-2458-3.
2. Tender GC, Serban D. Minimally invasive transforaminal lumbar interbody fusion: comparison of two techniques. Chirurgia (Bucur). 2014;109:812–21.
3. Wang J, et al. Comparison of one-level minimally invasive and open transforaminal lumbar interbody fusion in degenerative and isthmic spondylolisthesis grades 1 and 2. Eur Spine J. 2010;19:1780–4. https://doi.org/10.1007/s00586-010-1404-z.
4. Lee KH, Yue WM, Yeo W, Soeharno H, Tan SB. Clinical and radiological outcomes of open versus minimally invasive transforaminal lumbar interbody fusion. Eur Spine J. 2012;21:2265–70. https://doi.org/10.1007/s00586-012-2281-4.
5. Parker SL, et al. Minimally invasive versus open transforaminal lumbar interbody fusion for degenerative spondylolisthesis: comparative effectiveness and cost-utility analysis. World Neurosurg. 2014;82:230–8. https://doi.org/10.1016/j.wneu.2013.01.041.
6. Terman SW, et al. Minimally invasive versus open transforaminal lumbar interbody fusion: comparison of clinical outcomes among obese patients. J Neurosurg Spine. 2014;20:644–52. https://doi.org/10.3171/2014.2.SPINE13794.
7. Phan K, Hogan JA, Mobbs RJ. Cost-utility of minimally invasive versus open transforaminal lumbar interbody fusion: systematic review and economic evaluation. Eur Spine J. 2015;24:2503–13. https://doi.org/10.1007/s00586-015-4126-4.
8. Phan K, Rao PJ, Kam AC, Mobbs RJ. Minimally invasive versus open transforaminal lumbar interbody fusion for treatment of degenerative lumbar disease: systematic review and meta-analysis. Eur Spine J. 2015;24:1017–30. https://doi.org/10.1007/s00586-015-3903-4.
9. Goldstein CL, Macwan K, Sundararajan K, Rampersaud YR. Perioperative outcomes and adverse events of minimally invasive versus open posterior lumbar fusion: meta-analysis and systematic review. J Neurosurg Spine. 2016;24:416–27. https://doi.org/10.3171/2015.2.SPINE14973.
10. Virdee JS, Nadig A, Anagnostopoulos G, George KJ. Comparison of peri-operative and 12-month lifestyle outcomes in minimally invasive transforaminal lumbar interbody fusion versus conventional lumbar fusion. Br J Neurosurg. 2017;31:167. https://doi.org/10.1080/02688697.2016.1199790.
11. Wang HL, et al. Minimally invasive lumbar interbody fusion via MAST quadrant retractor versus open surgery: a prospective randomized clinical trial. Chin Med J. 2011;124:3868–74.
12. Serban D, Calina N, Tender G. Standard versus minimally invasive transforaminal lumbar interbody fusion: a prospective randomized study. Biomed Res Int. 2017;2017:7236970. https://doi.org/10.1155/2017/7236970.
13. Lee KH, Yeo W, Soeharno H, Yue WM. Learning curve of a complex surgical technique: minimally invasive transforaminal lumbar interbody fusion (MIS TLIF). J Spinal Disord Tech. 2014;27:E234–40. https://doi.org/10.1097/bsd.0000000000000089.

Chapter 7
Lateral Lumbar Interbody Fusion

Gabriel Tender, Daniel Serban, Niki Calina, Mihaela Florea, and Lindsay Lasseigne

Indications

Minimally invasive lateral retroperitoneal transpsoas approach for lumbar interbody fusion, or shortly Lateral Lumbar Interbody Fusion (LLIF) is the fastest growing type of minimally invasive spinal fusion in the United States.

The common indications for LLIF include:

- Segmental instability with grade 1 or 2 spondylolisthesis
- Segmental instability after previous laminectomy and/or discectomy
- Severe degenerative disc disease with resultant low back pain, with or without radiculopathy, after failure of conservative treatment
- Severe degenerative disease with latero-listhesis and/or focal scoliosis

Electronic Supplementary Material The online version of this chapter https://doi.org/10.1007/978-3-319-71943-6_7. contains supplementary material, which is available to authorized users.

G. Tender (✉)
Louisiana State University, New Orleans, LA, USA

D. Serban • N. Calina • M. Florea
Department of Neurosurgery, "Bagdasar-Arseni" Hospital, Bucharest, Romania

L. Lasseigne
Department of Neurosurgery, Louisiana State University Health Sciences Center, New Orleans, LA, USA
e-mail: llasse@lsuhsc.edu

G. Tender (ed.), *Minimally Invasive Spine Surgery Techniques*,
https://doi.org/10.1007/978-3-319-71943-6_7

Contraindications

Contraindications for this technique include:

- Grade 3 or 4 spondylolisthesis
- Anterior location of the femoral nerve, as seen on the axial MR images, particularly at the L4–5 level
- Previous retroperitoneal operations resulting in scarring

This technique can be applied in the lumbar spine at L4–5 and above, and in the thoracic spine below T5.

Most of the morbidity of this procedure comes from the transpsoas approach. Two conceptually different LLIF psoas dissection techniques can be used. One involves reliance on EMG and X-rays for correct placement of the tubular retractor, whereas the other relies on X-rays for the placement of an initial outer retractor on the surface of the psoas, followed by dissection of the psoas under direct visualization for placement of the second inner retractor. Once the lateral aspect of the annulus fibrosus is exposed, the discectomy and interbody cage placement is similar with both techniques.

Preoperative Planning

Common imaging modalities used preoperatively include MRI, dynamic X-rays, and CT scan.

The MRI is the most important preoperative study. Sagittal images provide information on the disc height, dimensions of the spinal canal and degree of stenosis, and status of the posterior elements. Axial images show the position of the femoral nerve in relation to the lateral aspect of the disc, the position of the large vessels, and the presence of possible retroperitoneal scarring.

The lateral X-rays show the height of the iliac crest in report to the L4–5 disc and should be done in all cases anticipating an L4–5 fusion. If the iliac crests projection, on a true lateral image, is above the midbody of L4, we recommend using an alternative approach (ALIF or MI TLIF), since the lateral approach, even with angled instruments, will be very difficult. The flexion-extension imaging shows possible dynamic instability. Standing scoliosis films may be necessary if deformity is suspected.

The CT scan may provide additional information on the bony anatomy (endplate changes, osteophytes, previous laminectomy, pedicle size etc), but is not mandatory for the preoperative work-up in most cases.

A DEXA scan can be done in patients suspected to have osteoporosis.

Surgical Technique

The following operative steps are described:

- patient positioning
- skin incision and bone marrow aspiration

- psoas dissection, EMG based
- psoas dissection under direct visualization
- discectomy
- cage insertion
- lateral plating
- closure
- patient repositioning
- percutaneous pedicle screw insertion

Patient Positioning

Correct patient positioning is critical, particularly in obese individuals. The patient is initially placed supine on the operating table for endotracheal intubation. A draw sheet under the patient is used to roll him 90°, in lateral decubitus position, usually with the left side up (due to the advantageous position of the great vessels when approaching from the left). A beanbag is NOT used for stabilization, as it may interfere with the lateral fluoroscopy. The back of the patient should be positioned at about 5 in. from the edge of the table, so that the table rail does not overlap with the lumbar spine on lateral fluoroscopy. A chest roll is placed in the patient's axilla. Patient's head is brought back towards the edge of the table, and the anesthesiologist typically inserts 2 or 3 folded sheets under the patients' head to keep it level with the rest of the body. Patient's arms are folded at the elbows; a folded pillow is placed between the bed and the lower hand, and another folded pillow is placed between patient's forearms, with the endotracheal tube fitting in the fold of the pillow. This position is maintained with tape starting anteriorly at the corner of the table and rolling over the patients forearm and shoulder to the other side of the table. Once the head and arms are in proper position, attention is turned towards immobilizing the thorax and pelvis in adequate position. The natural tendency is for the thorax to roll forward; therefore, with the assistant maintaining the thorax and hips in true lateral position, several rolls of tape are used to stabilize the patient to the table at the levels of the hip as well as upper thorax. We start with 3-in. silk tape at the edge of the table, on the rail anterior to the hips, go on the hips right below the iliac crest (without any protective towels!), then continue to the posterior rail, go under the table, and then continue one more time over the hips and to the posterior table rail. The same process is repeated at the thorax level, this time protecting the nipple. A final taping in a "figure-of-8" can be done, starting longitudinally at the level of the left hip, go caudally along the left thigh (protecting the fibular notch to prevent a peroneal injury), go to the anterior rail, under the table, and posterior rail, then along the calf in a caudal-cranial direction, and ending at the anterior rail (Fig. 7.1). This final taping also helps in obese patients by placing some tension on the lateral flank skin and making the incision easier.

The patient's hip joint should be placed at the level where the table can be flexed, in case further exposure of the L4–5 level is needed. Patient's legs are placed in slight flexion with a pillow in between the knees.

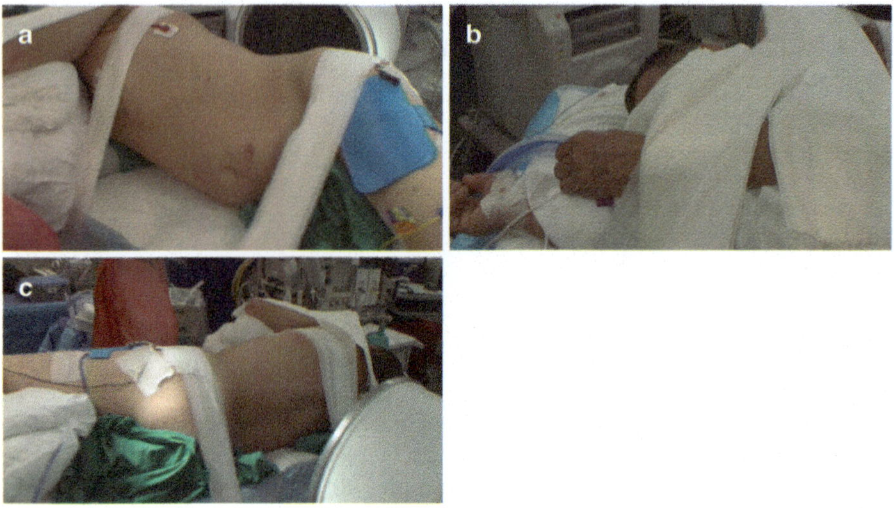

Fig. 7.1 Patient positioning. (**a**) and (**b**) Anterior view: the arms are flexed with pillows under and in between them. (**c**) Posterior view: the chest and hips are double-taped to the table

The first fluoroscopic image to be obtained is the AP. The table, not the C-arm, is tilted until the spinous process of the level of interest is exactly in the midline between the two corresponding pedicles. The C-arm is then switched to the lateral position, and the bed usually has to be placed in slight Trendelenburg position in order to achieve a true lateral image, with the two pedicles of the level of interest overlapping perfectly and each endplate appearing as a single line.

Skin Incision and Bone Marrow Aspiration

After this, the projection of the disc of interest is marked on the skin as guided by the lateral fluoroscopic image. This is typically just above the iliac crest for the L3–4 disc, and at the level of the crest for L4–5. Of course, if the L4–5 projection is below the crest, the skin incision should still be made at the top of the crest.

The skin incision follows the skin mark as described above and is typically about 3 cm in length. After local coagulation, the incision is extended through the superficial fascia, but not deeper.

We prefer to aspirate bone marrow from the anterior iliac crest at this time. From the anterior corner of the skin incision, the fascia is followed caudally to its' insertion on the iliac crest. The Jamshidi needle is then inserted into the crest as anterior as possible, where the crest is thicker. If actual cancellous graft is needed, we recommend harvesting it through an anterior, separate skin incision, as the crest is too thin in its' midportion (at the level of our skin incision) to be used for autologous graft harvesting.

Once the fascia is sharply open under the skin incision, the three muscles to be dissected (external oblique, internal oblique, and transversalis) follow three different directions and can be felt with the tip of the finger as the dissection is bluntly performed. Once the transversalis fascia is penetrated, a "pop" sensation is felt and the tip of the finger palpates a loose areolar tissue, which is the retroperitoneal fat. The finger is swiped over posteriorly over the quadratus lumborum muscle, and the retroperitoneal content is moved anteriorly. I prefer to insert two and then three fingers through the lateral abdominal wall opening, in order to make it easier to insert the tubular dilators and retractor. The blunt retroperitoneal dissection is continued until the tip of the finger encounters the psoas muscle. At this time, the tip of the transverse process of the level of interest can also be felt posterior to the psoas muscle. The psoas dissection is then performed differently, depending on the system employed.

Transpsoas Approach, EMG Based

This is the originally described approach and involves placement of a thin probe through the psoas muscle, targeting the junction between the anterior two thirds and the posterior third of the disc projection on lateral X-ray. The thin probe has directional electric conductivity, so that the base of the probe can be connected to a stimulating electrode and EMG recording from specific muscle groups determines the proximity of the motor nerve to the tip of the probe. Recorded values of 10 mA or above are considered safe, whereas values of 3 mA or less suggest direct contact between the tip of the probe and the motor (femoral) nerve. We prefer to place the small probe as far posterior as allowed by neuromonitoring, i.e., until values close to 10 mA are obtained upon stimulation. If this value is achieved while the tip of the probe is still too anterior, then the probe is pulled out of the psoas muscle and reinserted at a more anterior point, but with a more anterior-to-posterior angulation (the idea being to place a few more muscle fascicles between the tip of the probe and the nerve). The femoral nerve originates from the L2, L3, and L4 spinal nerves and is typically located posteriorly, close the neural foramina, but can be occasionally be found as far anterior as the middle of the disc projection, particularly at L4–5.

Once the small probe is placed in the best possible position (as far posterior as possible, while still recording over 10 mA), the C-arm is moved cranially and a Kirschner wire is placed through the probe into the soft disc. The position is verified again with fluoroscopy, to make sure the probe did not slip in a different position (since the disc feels like a hill, more prominent than the vertebral bodies above and below, the probe can easily slip cranially or caudally, particularly during the stimulation, when the contractions tend to move the probe). Sequentially larger diameter dilator tubes are then placed over the initial probe, and then a tubular retractor of appropriate length is sled over the tubes and then locked to the side of the table in the desired position via a rigid arm.

One of the most frustrating situations arises when the second and especially the third dilator yield a response at values less than 10 mA, sometimes as low as 5 mA. In these cases, we pull out the dilators and the pin, and reinsert at a more anterior point, but with a more anterior-to-posterior angulation, and try to start at a higher response with the small probe (e.g., 15 mA), anticipating that this response will get lower as the larger dilators are used. At the extreme, when the re-docking is performed by going anterior to the psoas muscle, this technique becomes the OLIF.

The tubular retractor typically has several parts that can be retracted in order to provide a larger field of view. Once the position of the retractor is confirmed with fluoroscopy and the exposed field is free of motor nerves (as tested by EMG direct stimulation), the retractor blades can be further stabilized either by a shim going into the disc space or by small screws going through the cranial and/or caudal blades and into the vertebral body. At this point the lateral aspect of the annulus fibrosus should be apparent. Sometimes, a small amount of muscle fibers remain between the tip of the retractor and the disc and can be easily dissected away with a Penfield 4 (but NOT with the Bovie cautery). Bleeding from small veins can be controlled with bipolar cautery, if necessary.

Transpsoas Approach Under Direct Visualization

This approach was more recently described and we used it with good results [1]. After the blunt dissection of the lateral wall muscles is completed, a tubular dilator is placed under fluoroscopic guidance targeting the junction between the anterior third and posterior two-thirds of the lateral disc projection. This is in contrast with the EMG technique, which targets a more posterior point. The tubular dilator is also guided with the finger, but its' tip is placed on the surface, and not through, the psoas muscle. A second and third dilators allow for placement of an appropriate length outer retractor that also rests on the surface of the psoas. After lateral fluoroscopy confirmation of adequate position, blunt psoas dissection under direct visualization (operative microscope or loupes) is performed with Penfield 4 and blunt Cobb instruments. Once the disc is encountered, gentle opening of the dissecting tools allow for exposure of the annulus fibrosus and placement of the independent inner retractor blades that will maintain the exposure for the remainder of the case. The inner retractor blades are stabilized either to directly to the table, or via a rigid ring to the outer retractor, which in turn is locked to the side of the table. Final imaging should confirm the adequate placement of the inner retractor blades. This technique has the potential advantage of protecting both motor and sensory nerves, since it does not directly rely on neuromonitoring. If the femoral nerve is encountered in the depth of the exposure, the inner retractor blades are repositioned, if possible (Video 7.1). Alternatively, the inner retractor is removed (or not inserted) and the outer retractor is moved more anteriorly on the surface of the psoas before muscle dissection is performed again.

Discectomy

Regardless of the system used for psoas dissection, once the retractor blades are in place, the lateral aspect of the annulus fibrosus is exposed. (This approach can also be used for removal of a far lateral disc herniation (Video 7.2), but the docking in those cases is obviously further posterior.) The surgeon should now see the highest point of the curve of the lateral aspect of the disc, and typically the discectomy is centered on this point. The annulotomy must be 22 mm in length in order to accommodate the standard size implant. If more space is needed in the exposure, it is usually easiest to continue the dissection anteriorly and place a retractor against the anterior longitudinal ligament (ALL); however, caution must be exercised at the time of implant (or trial) insertion, so that this doesn't slip anterior to the ALL into the great vessels. The location of the annulotomy (central versus more anterior) is very important, since the trials and eventually the cage will follow the space created by the annulotomy and discectomy.

Once the 22 mm annulotomy is performed, the disc material is removed with a combination of Cobb dissectors, rasps, and curettes. We prefer not to use disc shavers, since they can damage the endplates by creating a circular rather than square discectomy. Sometimes, the disc space is so narrow that it can only be accessed, initially, with a blunt Cobb; once the disc direction is established, rasps and sharp Cobb dissectors can complete the discectomy subsequently. We insert several trials of increasing height, pushing the dislodged disc material towards the bottom part of the disc, which facilitates its' removal with pituitary rongeurs (if not removed, this disc material will prevent the trial and/or cage from being inserted all the way to the other edge of the disc). Once most of the disc material is removed, the contralateral annulus is penetrated with a sharp Cobb under live AP fluoroscopic guidance; the tip of the Cobb has to go about 1 cm past the edge of the vertebral body.

Cage Insertion

The height and length of the interbody implant can be determined based on trials. We prefer to trial to a slightly less height than the cage (e.g., we trial to 11 mm height when planning to insert a 12 mm-height cage). We also prefer to insert the cage in between two "sliding" blades, in order to protect the endplates as well as keep the graft inside the cage.

Regarding cage insertion, several characteristics are important.

- Height. We prefer to use implants (filled with autologous bone or fusion extenders) with the height 2–3 mm larger than the original disc height; this allows for indirect decompression of the canal and posterior elements, without predisposing the construct to subsidence.
- Length. The choice of implant length depends on multiple factors, but we typically use implants that are contained within the disc space and not overhanging

on both sides, as some surgeons prefer. It has been shown that fusion rates correlate with the width, rather than the length, of the cage.

- Width. We use almost exclusively 22 mm-wide cages, with the 19 mm-wide cages reserved for the rare cases in which the femoral nerve is in the way or the anatomy is not favorable (Video 7.2). We have not used 26 mm-wide cages, but these may be appropriate for large-size individuals.
- Position. It is important to remember that the position of the cage in the disc space is determined at the time we make the annulotomy. Once the annulotomy and discectomy/endplate preparation are complete, the cage will follow the space created and cannot be adjusted to a more anterior or posterior position. Most cages are inserted around the center of the disc (the "50 yard line") or slightly anterior to it. This allows for good foraminal (indirect) decompression and some restoration of lordosis. However, if restoration of lordosis is the primary goal, we place the cage as anterior as possible (without disrupting the ALL) and later compress on the pedicle screws. We have not performed ALL release (which would enhance the achieved lordosis even further) since the risks of this maneuver have not been fully established.
- Dynamic (expandable) cages. The advantage of expandable cages is obvious—ease of insertion and ease of lordosis restoration (as much as the anterior longitudinal ligament permits). The downside is that, once the cage is expanded, the graft material may become loose and, according to Wolff's law, fusion rates may decrease. Therefore, in these cases, we recommend inserting more graft, preferably through the cage, after expansion (aka "backfill" of the cage).

After cage insertion, hemostasis can be achieved with Gelfoam and/or Surgiflo. Before removing the retractor, we always check to make sure the bottom of the cage is below the edge of the disc and the hemostasis is pristine. Final AP and lateral images are obtained to confirm the correct position and copious irrigation with antibiotic solution is performed.

Lateral Plating

We occasionally use lateral plating (as opposed to percutaneous pedicle screws) in patients with collapsed disc space and low degree of instability. Placement of a lateral plate requires slightly more cranio-caudal exposure, which may be difficult at L4–5. Moreover, we always use 4-screw plates, since the 2-screw plates are biomechanically insufficient. Some systems allow the plate to be slid over a temporary pin attached to the center of the cage, thus facilitating alignment of the cage and plate. Before inserting any of the screws, we take a lateral image to make sure the plate is long enough and is in roughly adequate position. Then, we start with the anterior and caudal screw. A pilot hole is made with the high-speed drill, followed by an awl inserted at a slight anterior to posterior angle, followed by the screw; we try to stay parallel to the endplate when inserting the screw. We do not currently use a bicortical purchase, unless the patient is osteoporotic. The screw is left slightly proud, to allow for some mobility of the plate until the second screw is inserted. After one more lateral image confirmation, we insert the anterior and cranial screw, using the same technique. Finally, the posterior cranial and caudal screws are inserted straight down (with no anterior to posterior angulation) and all the screws are tightened down. Plating can be difficult at L4–5, when the caudal screws may have to angled caudally (because of the iliac crest height), and also in patients with large lateral osteophytes, in which the plate cannot be brought all the way down to the vertebral body unless the osteophytes are partially removed prior to plate placement.

Closure

The muscles revert to their initial position and we only close the fascia with 0 Vycril on a UR needle, followed by the skin (interrupted 3-0 Vycril for the hypodermis and 4-0 running Monocryl for the subcuticular layer).

Patient Repositioning

We use bilateral percutaneous pedicle screws in most cases. Some surgeons insert them in lateral decubitus position, in order to save time. We prefer re-positioning the patient in prone position. Thus, the stretcher is brought to the beside behind the patient, the tape is released at all levels, and the patient is allowed to roll back on the side of the OR table and then slid onto the stretcher. The OR table is cleaned and two chest rolls are placed on it, covered by a draw sheet. The patient is then rolled onto the OR table in prone position.

Percutaneous Pedicle Screws

The patient is placed in prone position with the arms tucked to the sides and with adequate padding for all pressure points.

The accurate placement of the pedicle screws is dependent of the quality of the radiologic images. Therefore, obtaining true AP and lateral images prior to skin incision is of utmost importance.

The AP image should be obtained first. The C-arm is locked at 90°, perfectly centered on the vertebral body of interest. This is particularly important if the patient has significant deformity, in which case the C-arm should be readjusted for each vertebral body. The spinous process of the vertebral body of interest should be centered between the two pedicle rings; otherwise, the table (NOT the C-arm) should be tilted left or right until the desired position is achieved. Then, the table is placed either in Trendelenburg or reverse Trendelenburg until the superior endplate of the vertebral body of interest becomes a single line.

The lateral image is obtained next. If the AP image was perfect, now the posterior margin of the targeted vertebral body should appear as a single line. The perfect lateral image is obtained by "wagging" the C-arm until the two pedicles of the vertebral body of interest overlap. At this point, the superior and inferior endplates should also appear as a single line.

After this, the bony landmarks can be marked on patient's skin under AP fluoroscopy: the midline, the left and right pedicle lines, and the interpedicular line for the vertebral body of interest. The skin incision should be about 2 cm in length, vertical and centered on the interpedicular line, about 4–6 cm off the midline. This point is typically at or just lateral to the tip of the transverse process on the AP image. In large patients, the skin incision has to be made further lateral, in order to maintain the same lateral-to-medial angle of insertion.

The lumbar fascia is then incised with the knife medial to the skin incision. It is important to remember that the fascia is the layer that limits the exploration of the deep bony landmarks. Continuing in the same lateral to medial direction, the index finger can be inserted to find the junction between the transverse process and the lateral facet. Typically, the lateral facet is first encountered (since it is the most superficial), and then the finger is allowed to slide lateral to it and land on the posterior aspect of the transverse process. If the incision is too small to accommodate a finger, the same landmarks can be identified with the tip of a Jamshidi needle, with the aid of frequent fluoroscopic images. The ideal docking point is at the junction of the transverse process with the lateral facet, as medial as allowed by the lateral facet. On the AP image, this point will appear just outside the pedicle ring; if it appears inside the pedicle ring, it is likely that the tip of the needle is actually riding high on the lateral facet, not on the transverse process. On the lateral image, the tip of the needle should be just above the ring of the transverse process, not high on the lateral facet, and the trajectory should pass through the pedicle, parallel to the endplates. If fine adjustments are necessary, the tip of the Jamshidi needle can be moved with both hands (for maximal control) in millimeter increments, on the base of the transverse process, until the desired position is achieved.

Once the correct docking point is obtained, the needle is gently tapped through the pedicle. For the lower lumbar pedicles, the direction is typically lateral to medial and cranial to caudal, but the angles vary with each level. As the needle is advanced through the pedicle, there should be no increased resistance (that would signify cortical bone and therefore imminent pedicle wall breach). The most important images are obtained when the tip of the needle reaches the base of the pedicle on the lateral image; at this time, the tip of the needle should be still within the pedicle ring on the AP image.

At this time, neuromonitoring is usually employed. The shaft of the needle is stimulated, and a response of 10 mA or above signifies that the medial or inferior pedicle walls have not been breached.

A particular situation is encountered if the tip of the needle is very close to the medial border of the pedicle ring on the AP image, and neuromonitoring yields low responses (e.g., 4–7 mA). In this situation, it is likely that the needle has violated the lateral recess, which sometimes loops under the line of the pedicle ring. Therefore, it is recommended that the tip of the needle should be well within the pedicle ring on the AP images, when it reaches the base of the pedicle on the lateral images.

Another important technical tool is changing the direction of the Jamshidi needle while in the pedicle. Indeed, if the original trajectory is angled too much lateral to medial, and the tip of the needle gets too close to the medial border of the pedicle on the AP image, the angulation of the needle can be changed to a more straight trajectory, without withdrawing the needle from the pedicle. The angulation can also be changed in a cranio-caudal direction, in order to keep the needle parallel to the endplates. Beveled needles are particularly useful in this situation.

Once the needle trajectory is deemed safe, the tip of the needle is advanced into the vertebral body for a couple of centimeters, and then the center part of the needle is removed and a K-wire is inserted for about another centimeter past the tip of the Jamshidi needle, in order to stabilize it to the cancellous bone and make it less likely to inadvertently come out during the placement of the tap and screw. Then, the Jamshidi needle is removed, while the K-wire is kept in place with the other hand.

After this, most systems have a series of tubular dilators that slide over the K-wire; the outer dilator and the K-wire are kept in place, whereas the inner dilators are removed to make room for the tap and screw. The tap is then advanced over the K-wire into the pedicle of the vertebral body; it is sufficient (and recommended) to tap only past the base of the pedicle and not all the way into the vertebral body. For biomechanical reasons, we recommend undertapping by 2 mm (i.e., use a 4.5 mm tap for a 6.5 mm screw), in order to maintain the good purchase of the screw into the bone. It is important to maintain the direction of the K-wire with the tap; if the tap is not aligned with the K-wire, the part of the K-wire in the vertebral body starts to bend at the tip of the tap, and when a critical angle is reached, the tap cannot advance any more, and any further turns of the tap do nothing but strip (and destroy) the pedicle.

The tap is then removed and the screw (typically 6.5 × 45 mm for the average person) is inserted over the K-wire. Once the tip of the screw passes the base of the pedicle, the K-wire can be removed, and the screw further inserted through the previously created trajectory. The screw insertion must stop just before the head of the screw abuts the lateral facet; otherwise, the screw head loses its' poliaxial capabilities and makes subsequent rod insertion more difficult. All the screws have extender blades attached to their heads, in order to facilitate rod placement.

Of course, at least 2 pedicle screws per side have to be inserted. The described technique is changed in the fact that most surgeons choose to insert all the K-wires in their respective pedicles before performing the tapping and screw insertion. In patients requiring long constructs (e.g., for trauma fixation, or in deformity correction), it is extremely important to be consistent with the docking point for each level, since the junctions between the transverse process and the lateral facet are lined up in a cranio-caudal fashion.

Specific Levels

The L4–5 Level

This level is the most commonly treated as well as the most difficult to treat. Two elements are critical for feasibility: the iliac crest height and the femoral nerve position.

A preoperative true lateral X-ray is mandatory and will show the height of the iliac crest in rapport to the L4–5 disc. If the crest is below the disc, then the surgery can proceed without worries, similar to an L3–4 disc. If the crest projects at the midbody of L4, several adjustments can be made: the table can be flexed to open the L5–S1 disc and provide a little more exposure for L4–5; the skin incision can be made over the iliac crest edge and the finger dissection of the abdominal wall muscles can be forced right over the bony ridge of the iliac crest; appropriate angled instruments must be used for discectomy and implant insertion. If the crest projects higher than the L4 midbody, then a different approach (e.g., MI TLIF) should be used; however, this usually only happens in patients with transitional anatomy. Another option is to convert to the more anterior approach, i.e. the OLIF.

The femoral nerve position on the side of the disc can be determined on the axial T2-weighted MR images. The nerve appears as a dark shadow surrounded by white fat and is typically located posteriorly, close to the lumbar foramen. However, in about 25% of patients, it can be located as anterior as the middle of the lateral aspect of the disc. These cases should be identified preoperatively and an alternative route (e.g., MI TLIF or OLIF) should be used. Exposure and retraction of the femoral nerve in these cases is NOT recommended. If the nerve is encountered despite careful preoperative planning, an attempt can be made to insert the cage behind the femoral nerve (Video 7.3), although this is a risky and advanced technique.

The L3–4 Level

This is the second-most commonly treated level as well as the easiest to treat. In fact, we recommend starting with this level, when learning the LLIF technique. At this level, neither the iliac crest nor the ribs are in the way (hence no need for angled instruments). Moreover, the psoas muscle is thinner (thus easier to dissect) and the femoral nerve is located posteriorly (thus not endangered during the exposure). The standard technique described above applies to this level.

The L2–3 Level

This level may be difficult because the tip of the eleventh rib may be in the way. However, we recommend NOT removing the rib; sufficient exposure can be achieved going around it. Once the retroperitoneal space is accessed, the rest of the procedure is relatively easy, as the psoas muscle is thin and the femoral nerve (the L2 component) is not in the way.

The L1–2 Level

This level may be difficult because the surgeon must make the skin incision parallel to the ribs and dissect the intercostal muscles to gain access to the retropleural, not retroperitoneal, space. As the dissection is continued with the index finger between the inner side of the rib and the parietal pleura, eventually the vertebral body covered by the thin psoas muscle is encountered. The dilators and then the retractor are placed against the diaphragm dome, which will push the retroperitoneal content anteriorly. In order to access the L1–2 disc, a small opening in the diaphragm insertion must be made with the long bayoneted knife, and can be closed at the end of the case (although not mandatory). If the intercostal opening is not lined up with the disc, angled instruments must be used occasionally.

Pearls and Pitfalls

LLIF Versus MI TLIF

While the minimally invasive transforaminal lumbar interbody fusion (MI TLIF) is a great technique that can be applied to most patients with degenerative pathology, the LLIF offers certain advantages that make it a favorite in selected patients. We present below a synopsis of the usual patient presentations (assuming that they have already had unsuccessful maximal conservative treatment) and our selection process of LLIF versus MI TLIF.

At L3–4 and above, we prefer using the LLIF, since the MI TLIF is more difficult and dangerous. Even if there is a disc herniation with a free fragment, we perform the LLIF first, then use a minimally invasive retractor to perform a laminectomy and disc fragment removal, followed by pedicle screw insertion through the same incision.

At L4–5, both techniques can be used, and below we present our selection process.

In patients with low-grade spondylolisthesis and preserved disc height, with or without resultant central or lateral recess stenosis, but without a disc herniation/extrusion, we prefer using the LLIF, because it offers superior biomechanical support and fusion surface. If the patient has a large disc herniation/extruded free fragment, we prefer using the MI TLIF, because it offers direct decompression of the nerve by removing the extruded fragment (this fragment cannot be influenced by the ligamentotaxis, which LLIF relies on, in part, for the indirect decompression).

In patients with severe collapse of the disc space, both LLIF and MI TLIF work well and the choice is usually based on other anatomical factors (e.g., the iliac crest height) and surgeons' preference.

In patients with post-laminectomy instability, we prefer using the LLIF, in order to avoid the posterior midline scarring.

In patients with single-level focal scoliosis, we prefer using the LLIF approaching from the convex side; this provides easy access to the disc and excellent correction of the deformity by the simple insertion of the interbody implant.

In patients with multi-level degenerative lumbar scoliosis, we prefer starting with LLIF at all the affected levels (usually 3 or 4) approaching from the concave side (since it requires less abdominal wall and psoas muscle dissection for the multiple levels), followed by percutaneous screw/rod fixation. It is important to remember that the lateral fusion is only FDA approved for one or two levels.

In obese patients with operative pathology, we prefer using the LLIF when possible, since the abdominal fat falls forward in lateral decubitus and the access to the spine is a lot easier than in the MI TLIF approach.

Discectomy and Endplate Preparation

Since the discs have a bi-convex shape (unless severely degenerated, in which case they become flat), endplate preparation must be done respecting its' concave shape. The best preparation, in our opinion, is done with a wide Cobb (20 or 22 mm) that follows the dissection plane between the disc and the endplate. As the Cobb follows the concave surface of the endplate, the direction of the shaft changes from cranially angled (initially) to straight (as the tip of the Cobb passes the midpoint of the disc). If this direction is not changed, there is a risk of endplate and vertebral body violation in the deep (contralateral) half of the vertebral body.

Stand-Alone LLIF

Most patients undergoing LLIF should have some type of posterior stabilization. The preferred method of most surgeons is the percutaneous pedicle screw/rod fixation, whether unilateral or bilateral. Others have used facet screws or facet dowels.

In selected patients, stand-alone LLIF can also be used. The typical candidate cannot tolerate long operations, but has reasonably good quality bone (i.e., is not severely osteoporotic), no spondylolisthesis, and a collapsed (and sometimes sclerotic) disc space. In these cases, we insert slightly longer cages, extending 1–2 mm beyond the edges of the vertebral body, and we keep the patient in a TLSO brace for 3 months postoperatively.

Spondylolisthesis

These cases are more difficult because there is less disc available for annulotomy and cage insertion, particularly for grade 2 spondylolisthesis (grade 3 and 4 are contraindications, for the same reason). Occasionally, we use 19 mm-width cages in these cases. Once the cage is inserted, particularly if the disc was collapsed, the spondylolisthesis is already partially reduced. The case is finished by using the percutaneous pedicle screw reduction system to complete the realignment.

Previous Discectomy

These cases can be done with no changes from the standard technique, since no scar is encountered during the exposure. One potential concern, particularly in patients who had the discectomy recently, is for the graft to extrude through the posterior annular defect into the spinal canal. However, since the graft is only placed inside the cage and not in front of it, this risk is fairly small.

Previous TLIF

These cases can also be done with no changes from the standard technique, until the time of discectomy. Since the TLIF cage is likely loose (since the re-intervention is done for pseudarthrosis), the surgeon can attempt to remove it in one piece with dedicated instruments (Fig. 7.2). If this is not possible, we have used the high-speed drill or osteotomes to break the cage and remove it in several pieces with the pituitary rongeurs. The rest of the case (discectomy, endplate preparation, LLIF cage insertion) is performed using the normal technique.

Collapsed Disc

When the disc is almost completely collapsed, or when there is a shell of calcification or cortical bone covering the annulus, it may be difficult to access the disc. In these cases, we use the high-speed drill to uncover the "entrance" into the disc, over a distance of 22 mm, sufficient to permit the insertion of a blunt Cobb. Care must be exercised not to go to deep with the Cobb from the first pass, as it may be difficult to pull out. Therefore, we insert the Cobb about a third of the disc at the time, then pull out and reinsert deeper, until the other side of the disc is reached.

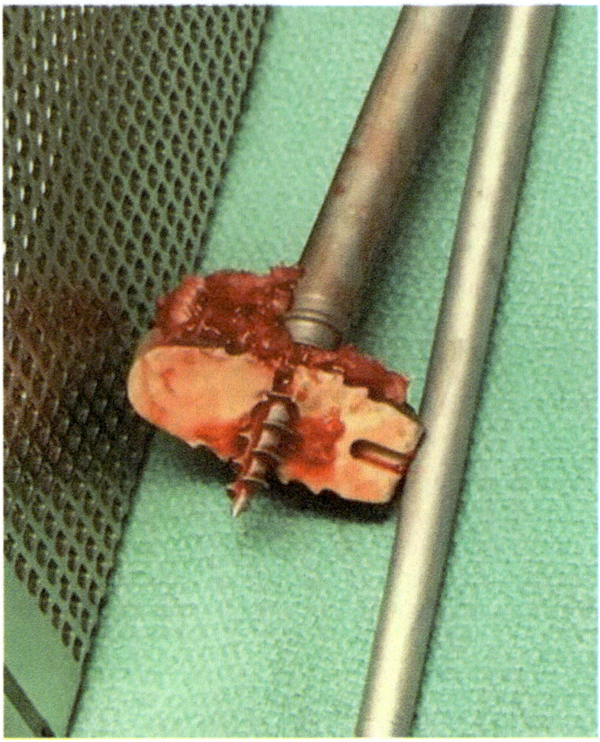

Fig. 7.2 TLIF cage removed via the lateral approach, still attached to the remover

Normal Height Disc

These are typically patients with bilateral pars defects and grade 1 or 2 spondylolisthesis, but with preserved disc height and often with large disc herniations. In these cases, we try to insert 22 mm-width cages (rather than 19 mm) to maximize the fusion surface (since we are asking the bone to grow over a longer distance, between the endplates). Also, since there are bilateral pars defects, it is easy to overdistract; therefore, we insert the cage that feels slightly snug (usually 14 or 15 mm in height) and then compress on the percutaneous pedicle screws in the second part of the procedure.

Penetration of Contralateral Annulus

When the tip of the Cobb reaches the contralateral annulus, it usually has a bouncy feel, unless the disc is severely collapsed and degenerated. In order to penetrate the annulus without going too far into the contralateral psoas, we recommend holding the Cobb from the shaft, just above the retractor, and apply low-force taps until the tip of the Cobb goes through.

The other concern when penetrating the annulus is injury to the contralateral femoral nerve. This occurs if the trajectory of the discectomy is oblique from anterior to posterior, whether planned or accidental. Perfect positioning and frequent lateral fluoroscopic imaging can prevent this complication.

Two-Level LLIF

Most commonly, this is done at L3–4 and L4–5. In these cases, the lateral abdominal wall can be either opened over a wider distance (similar to the exposure for a corpectomy) or two separate entries through the lateral wall can be made. It is a mistake to try to make a single small lateral wall opening in between the two discs and then try to forcefully mobilize the retractor from one disc to the other, as the lateral wall is rigid and the retractor will end up in an angled position at both discs, making the discectomy and cage insertion more difficult than it needs to be.

Multi-Level LLIF

Most commonly, this is done between L1 and L5 in patients with deformity (i.e., scoliosis). This application is not FDA approved, since the lateral fusion is only indicated for one or two levels. We prefer performing the approach on the concave side, since not only the skin incision is smaller (as all the disc lines converge around the same spot on the lateral abdominal wall) but also the L4–5 and sometimes L3–4 discs cannot be accessed from the convex side. The psoas dissection is also limited on the concave side, as the vertebral bodies are collapsed on the concave side of the deformity. Finally, we perform the LLIFs from cranial to caudal, since the insertion of the cage reduces the deformity and, if we started at the caudal level, the cranial levels would become inaccessible through the same skin incision. The insertion of the LLIF cages already partially corrects the scoliosis; the percutaneous pedicles screws and rods complete the deformity correction. This indication is not FDA approved for the lateral approach.

Femoral Nerve in the Way

If the preoperative MRI was adequately interpreted, the femoral nerve should not be encountered in an anterior position. However, occasionally, the MRI can be misinterpreted, and a small amount of what appears to be just fat (white on the T2-weighted images) and with no grey structure to suggest the femoral nerve in it, may actually harbor the nerve. In these cases, we recommend trying to find a window for the annulotomy and discectomy in front or, more rarely, behind the nerve (Video 7.2). If this is not feasible, we recommend aborting the case and using an alternate route to perform the fusion.

Anterior Longitudinal Ligament Release

We have not performed ALL release yet, since the safety of this procedure has not been established. Nonetheless, some surgeons use the ALL release and hyperlordotic cages to increase the length of the anterior column and correct kyphosis or insufficient lordosis. These cages come with a stabilization screw, which prevents them to slip anteriorly and damage the great vessels. Posterior instrumentation is mandatory.

Complications

Nerve Injury

There are several nerves at risk during this procedure and the subsequent pain syndromes have been well described.

In the lateral abdominal wall, the ilioinguinal and iliohypogastric nerves travel in between the oblique muscles. Therefore, dissection of these muscles must be done bluntly, rather than with the knife or Bovie cautery.

On the anterior aspect of the quadratus lumborum and towards the pelvic ring, the lateral femoral cutaneous nerve can be injured during the retroperitoneal dissection. Since this is typically done with the index finger, the surgeon should avoid breaking any "stringy" structure that may be a nerve.

The genitofemoral nerve surfaces on the psoas muscle at the L3–4 level and has a variable position at the L4–5 level. This is the nerve best protected by the direct visualization technique, since it is a sensory nerve and is not detectable by neuromonitoring. It has been our experience that the genitofemoral nerve is often in the way of the transpsoas exposure (Videos 7.4 and 7.5) and, if not visualized (as in the EMG-based technique), can likely be injured.

The femoral nerve is the most important and its injury results not only in sensory, but also motor deficits. This nerve can be injured both directly and indirectly, by stretching it over a long period of time with either the posterior retractor blade and/or by breaking the table too much and putting the psoas muscle and femoral nerve under tension. Neurostimulation at the time of retractor insertion as well as continuous EMG monitoring are used to detect and decrease the injury to this nerve.

Cage Retropulsion

This complication is rare and involves delayed migration of a cage laterally, along its' insertion path. In these cases, if symptomatic, the cage can be re-exposed and either removed or reinserted, this time preferably replaced with an expandable version and/or blocked with a lateral plate.

Subsidence and Vertebral Body Fractures

This is probably an under-reported complication. In patients with osteoporosis, we recommend using the widest cage possible and supplement with bilateral pedicle screws. If symptomatic subsidence or vertebral body fractures occur, posterior instrumentation over one or several segments is usually indicated [2].

Massive Bleeding

This is a rare, but potentially devastating, complication [3]. If injury of the great vessels occurs, we recommend temporary tamponade and emergent consultation of the vascular or general surgeon. Occasionally, the vascular injury can be repaired by endovascular stenting, rather than open repair or ligation.

Pseudarthrosis

With proper technique, very few patients should experience this complication. The treatment consists in adding a postero-lateral and posterior fusion, possibly adding (off-label) rhBMP.

Adjacent Level Disease

This is a delayed complication that typically occurs 5–10 years after the original surgery. If the L5–S1 level is involved, we recommend revising with a stand-alone ALIF, unless contraindicated. If L3–4 of above levels are involved, we recommend using additional LLIF cages.

Literature Review

This technique has been extensively covered in the recent years' literature.

Initial studies focused on the feasibility of this approach and the range of complications [4–10]. Davis et al. found that the proximity of the neural elements to the L4–5 disc space will almost always lead to their displacement during the procedure [5] and Banagan et al. showed that there is no absolute safe zone when performing the procedure from L1–L5 [6].

Subsequent studies evaluated the specific complication profile [1, 11, 12] and the long-term results [13–17] of this approach. Youssef et al. found a low complication rate and high arthrodesis rate in a retrospective chart review [7]. A retrospective review by Cahill et al. also showed a low complication rate, with a 4.8% rate of femoral nerve injury at L4–5 and 0% at higher levels. However, Joseph et al. performed a meta analysis that showed a 9.4% rate of transient motor deficit, 2.5% permanent motor deficit and a 27.1% rate of sensory deficits [18]. In comparison to the ALIF, a meta-analysis by Hartl et al. found a higher rate of neurologic complications (but lower overall complication rate) due to lumbar plexus injuries [19].

Recent literature has focused on the expansion of indications for this technique [20, 21] and further refinement of outcomes [22–24]. It has utility in trauma, osteodiscitis and deformity surgery (with correction of upwards of 20° of coronal curvature reported in the literature) [25]. Long-term outcomes are generally good, with fusion rates approaching 90%.

Conclusion

The LLIF is an excellent option for selected patients and should be included in the armamentarium of every spine surgeon.

Addendum: Informative Letter to the Patients

The following informative letter is NOT intended to cover ALL the possible complications and scenarios. It is only intended to serve as a general guide, to improve patients' understanding of the operation.

This procedure can be very long. Despite careful padding of all pressure points, abrasions and pressure sores can occur. Generally these are minor, but can be serious, especially if they occur on the face. Nerve damage, particularly at the joints, can also occur. Blood clots forming in the legs, with potential death from spread to the lungs, are always a worry, and we use special inflatable devices to minimize that risk. Blood loss during this kind of surgery is normal and unavoidable, and sometimes we need to give transfusions from the blood bank. All of the blood is carefully tested, but unfortunately no test is perfect and there is always a small risk of acquiring some disease, such as hepatitis or AIDS. Death from anesthesia reaction or massive blood loss is possible, but fortunately extremely rare.

We make a one-inch skin incision on the side, just above the hip bone, usually on the left. Before we go through the abdominal wall, we use this incision to take a small amount of your bone marrow from the hip bone, to concentrate it and use it for the fusion. Rarely, you may experience pain and soreness at the site where bone marrow has been harvested. Damage to small nerves in the area can lead to numbness or even pain towards the thigh or groin area.

We then dissect the muscles in the abdominal wall to get to the abdominal cavity. Sometimes, this may cause pain and/or numbness in the groin or anterior thigh. Using our fingers, we then sweep the bowels and abdominal organs out of the way and reach the spinal column with a small retractor, under X-ray guidance. At this point, an operating microscope is used to allow us to keep the incision as small as possible, yet have excellent vision so we can see what needs to be done. In order to get to the spine, we have to go through a thick muscle called psoas. There are several nerves in this muscle. We try to protect these nerves by doing the dissection under direct visualization and also by recording any abnormal electric potentials that appear when the nerves are stimulated. Nonetheless, it is very common in the first 3 months after surgery to have pain and/or paresthesias over the thigh or groin. Sometimes, when the larger nerves are stretched or damaged, you may have weakness in the leg, especially when trying to straighten out your knee. While most of these changes resolve by 3 months after the surgery, sometimes they persist forever. Another potential complication (but fortunately very rare) is injury to the bowels, kidney, or large vessels; these may require opening the abdomen widely (usually by a general surgeon) and may result in serious damage and even death.

Once we get to the side of the spine, we then remove the bad disc or discs and prepare the area to accept the fusion construct. After we take out the disc, we replace it with a synthetic box we call "cage" that is filled up with bone graft and will promote the bony fusion. We are careful to avoid damage to the nerves in the spinal canal, which are very close to our "working area". However, such damage (while very rare) is a risk and can result in paralysis from nerve damage, loss of bowel, bladder, and sexual function, numbness, lack of feeling or sensation, or even severe pain below the waist. X-rays are used throughout the procedure to maximize the safety.

In order to give instant strength and stability to the spine and to increase the probability of the natural bony fusion healing properly, we use either a lateral plate (that can be inserted through the same incision) or screws and rods (that have to be inserted through two 1-in. incisions in the back). We place the screws accurately with the aid of intraoperative X-ray guidance. Nerve or blood vessel damage is possible, but fortunately quite rare. These devices function as an internal cast to keep the spinal bones immobile while the bone cells are forming the fusion mass. (If you're gluing two pieces of wood together, the glue is more likely to stick if you keep the wood pieces in a vice until the glue is set.) The screws and rods have been engineered and designed for endurance, but if a natural bony fusion does not form, eventually they will work loose or break. Another risk of any type of implanted foreign (non-natural) body is the possibility of infection. If this occurs (which is rare) it is early, and not months or years later. Generally removal of the screws is not necessary (to treat the infection), but prolonged antibiotics and debriding (cleaning up) procedures could be required.

It is important that you understand that this is a serious and possibly painful operation with a long and slow recovery. Most frequently, after the surgery you will be moved from the recovery room to a normal hospital room. Occasionally, if the surgery takes longer than a few hours, you may need to be monitored in the intensive care unit. Sometimes the intestines are sluggish for a few days and until you begin to "pass gas", your intake of food may be restricted. We encourage you to walk with assistance as soon as possible, and it is hoped that the total hospital stay will be in the range of 1–4 days. Of course, this is varied as needed on an individual basis.

At home we would encourage a program of walking on a level surface, gradually increasing the distance to between 2 and 3 miles a day. At about 3 months, a home exercise regimen can be cautiously started. Return to daily activities is highly variable, but in general it is sometimes possible to return to the equivalent of a light office type job at about that time (3 months). Maximal medical improvement is generally reached around a year after the date of surgery. It is generally not possible to engage in heavy manual labor type occupations following an operation of this nature.

Over the 6–12 months after surgery, it is hoped that the operated discs will heal and grow into a strong bony mass, so as to cause a solid union between the bones. This is a gradual process and at first there is no increased strength. This healing process is dependent upon the patient's powers of healing and does not always occur properly. The use of nicotine in any form (cigarettes, smokeless tobacco, nicotine patches, or nicotine gum) interferes with bone healing and dramatically decreases the odds of a successful fusion. You should not smoke or use nicotine in any form! Generally about 3 months is required for the fusion to begin to set, but strengthening continues for about a year or more. Also, for the first several months after surgery it is best to avoid non-steroidal anti-inflammatory drugs (such as aspirin, Motrin, Aleve, Naprosyn, etc.). These medications may interfere with bone healing. Tylenol use is OK, but you should be careful not to exceed the recommended dose. We expect to achieve a successful fusion for one disc level in about 90% and for two levels in about 80%. Sometimes postoperative X-rays show that the fusion has not healed to form solid bone. Most of the time, this does not seem to matter because a tough scar tissue-like gristle has formed instead and there are no symptoms. Occasionally, however, the failed fusion is symptomatic. That is called a pseudoarthrosis and repeat surgery is sometimes required. The type of surgery in those cases depends on individual circumstances.

Major complications (life threatening) may occur in about 2% of cases. The most common major complication is implant malposition or migration and may require reoperation. Sudden massive blood loss could occur, resulting in death. Other major complications include pneumonia and pulmonary embolism (blood clot going to the lungs).

There is also the chance that another type of fusion operation will be required if this one does not heal solidly. For example, it might be necessary to perform an additional operation in the back or front of the spine, with more bone graft added at that time.

One last potential problem after fusion surgery is what we call "juxtafusional disease". After you have had a successful spinal fusion, that segment becomes immobile and the joints above and/or below that fusion are subjected to increased stress. Over the years, these joints can have problems that may require further surgery.

It is very important to emphasize that no operation or device is a "spine transplant". Results on an individual basis cannot be predicted, and therefore we certainly cannot give any guarantees or promises. Once you have a bad back, you always will have a bad back to some degree. You could be no better, or even worse. Most patients indicate that *on average* the pain is improved from "marked" to "mild". While this is a great improvement, it is usually not improved to "occasional" or "none". Whether you will be able to return to their pre-injury or preoperative level of functioning will have to be determined on an individual basis. As a general rule, it is about a year before patients are "over" the operation because recovery and reconditioning is a slow process. It is sometimes necessary to call upon the Departments of Physical Medicine & Rehabilitation and Occupational Medicine to perform functional capacity evaluations (FCE) to determine a patient's actual limitations and abilities.

My general advice to anyone with a spinal affliction of this nature is to "live with it" (if possible). Of course that's easy for me to say because I'm not the one hurting. This operation has been recommended in the belief that your condition is serious and therefore taking the risks of surgery makes sense. I believe this is a good operation that is the best choice for your particular problem. If your only affliction is pain, the decision is yours and yours alone as to whether you can live with it. While I obviously hope and believe that this operation will help you, I cannot give any guarantees or promises about results. It is possible that you could be the same or even worse. Furthermore, my general recommendation is to "live with it" if possible and avoid the risks and uncertainties of surgery. Nevertheless I am offering my surgical services in an attempt to help you, but the decision to proceed is up to you.

References

1. Tender GC, Serban D. Genitofemoral nerve protection during the lateral retroperitoneal transpsoas approach. Neurosurgery. 2013;73:ons192–6; discussion ons196-197. https://doi.org/10.1227/01.neu.0000431473.49042.95.
2. Tender GC. Caudal vertebral body fractures following lateral interbody fusion in nonosteoporotic patients. Ochsner J. 2014;14:123–30.
3. Assina R, Majmundar NJ, Herschman Y, Heary RF. First report of major vascular injury due to lateral transpsoas approach leading to fatality. J Neurosurg Spine. 2014;21:794–8. https://doi.org/10.3171/2014.7.spine131146.
4. Guerin P, et al. Safe working zones using the minimally invasive lateral retroperitoneal transpsoas approach: a morphometric study. Surg Radiol Anat. 2011;33:665–71. https://doi.org/10.1007/s00276-011-0798-6.
5. Davis TT, Bae HW, Mok JM, Rasouli A, Delamarter RB. Lumbar plexus anatomy within the psoas muscle: implications for the transpsoas lateral approach to the L4-L5 disc. J Bone Joint Surg Am. 2011;93:1482–7. https://doi.org/10.2106/JBJS.J.00962.
6. Banagan K, Gelb D, Poelstra K, Ludwig S. Anatomic mapping of lumbar nerve roots during a direct lateral transpsoas approach to the spine: a cadaveric study. Spine (Phila Pa 1976). 2011;36:E687–91. https://doi.org/10.1097/BRS.0b013e3181ec5911.

7. Youssef JA, et al. Minimally invasive surgery: lateral approach interbody fusion: results and review. Spine (Phila Pa 1976). 2010;35:S302–11. https://doi.org/10.1097/BRS.0b013e3182023438.
8. Rodgers WB, Cox CS, Gerber EJ. Early complications of extreme lateral interbody fusion in the obese. J Spinal Disord Tech. 2010;23:393–7. https://doi.org/10.1097/BSD.0b013e3181b31729.
9. Jahangiri FR, et al. Protecting the genitofemoral nerve during direct/extreme lateral interbody fusion (DLIF/XLIF) procedures. Am J Electroneurodiagnostic Technol. 2010;50:321–35.
10. Knight RQ, Schwaegler P, Hanscom D, Roh J. Direct lateral lumbar interbody fusion for degenerative conditions: early complication profile. J Spinal Disord Tech. 2009;22:34–7. https://doi.org/10.1097/BSD.0b013e3181679b8a.
11. Cahill KS, Martinez JL, Wang MY, Vanni S, Levi AD. Motor nerve injuries following the minimally invasive lateral transpsoas approach. J Neurosurg Spine. 2012;17:227–31. https://doi.org/10.3171/2012.5.SPINE1288.
12. Ahmadian A, Deukmedjian AR, Abel N, Dakwar E, Uribe JS. Analysis of lumbar plexopathies and nerve injury after lateral retroperitoneal transpsoas approach: diagnostic standardization. J Neurosurg Spine. 2012. https://doi.org/10.3171/2012.11.SPINE12755.
13. Aichmair A, et al. Neurological deficits following lateral lumbar interbody fusion - a six year trend analysis of a single institution. Spine (Phila Pa 1976). 2013. https://doi.org/10.1097/BRS.0b013e3182a3d1b4.
14. Ahmadian A, et al. Minimally invasive lateral retroperitoneal transpsoas interbody fusion for L4-5 spondylolisthesis: clinical outcomes. J Neurosurg Spine. 2013. https://doi.org/10.3171/2013.6.SPINE1340.
15. Uribe JS, et al. Minimally invasive lateral approach for symptomatic thoracic disc herniation: initial multicenter clinical experience. J Neurosurg Spine. 2012;16:264–79. https://doi.org/10.3171/2011.10.SPINE11291.
16. Patel VC, Park DK, Herkowitz HN. Lateral transpsoas fusion: indications and outcomes. ScientificWorldJournal. 2012;2012:893608. https://doi.org/10.1100/2012/893608.
17. Malham GM, Ellis NJ, Parker RM, Seex KA. Clinical outcome and fusion rates after the first 30 extreme lateral interbody fusions. ScientificWorldJournal. 2012;2012:246989. https://doi.org/10.1100/2012/246989.
18. Joseph JR, Smith BW, La Marca F, Park P. Comparison of complication rates of minimally invasive transforaminal lumbar interbody fusion and lateral lumbar interbody fusion: a systematic review of the literature. Neurosurg Focus. 2015;39:E4. https://doi.org/10.3171/2015.7.focus15278.
19. Hartl R, Joeris A, McGuire RA. Comparison of the safety outcomes between two surgical approaches for anterior lumbar fusion surgery: anterior lumbar interbody fusion (ALIF) and extreme lateral interbody fusion (ELIF). Eur Spine J. 2016;25:1484–521. https://doi.org/10.1007/s00586-016-4407-6.
20. Ghobrial GM, Al-Saiegh F, Franco D, Benito D, Heller J. Lateral lumbar retroperitoneal transpsoas approach in the setting of spondylodiscitis: a technical note. J Clin Neurosci. 2017;39:193–8. https://doi.org/10.1016/j.jocn.2016.12.028.
21. Patel NB, Dodd ZH, Voorhies J, Horn EM. Minimally invasive lateral transpsoas approach for spinal discitis and osteomyelitis. J Clin Neurosci. 2015;22:1753–7. https://doi.org/10.1016/j.jocn.2015.03.061.
22. Sembrano JN, Tohmeh A, Isaacs R. Two-year comparative outcomes of MIS lateral and MIS transforaminal interbody fusion in the treatment of degenerative spondylolisthesis: part I: clinical findings. Spine (Phila Pa 1976). 2016;41(Suppl 8):S123–32. https://doi.org/10.1097/brs.0000000000001471.
23. Lehmen JA, Gerber EJ. MIS lateral spine surgery: a systematic literature review of complications, outcomes, and economics. Eur Spine J. 2015;24(Suppl 3):287–313. https://doi.org/10.1007/s00586-015-3886-1.
24. Berjano P, et al. Fusion rate following extreme lateral lumbar interbody fusion. Eur Spine J. 2015;24(Suppl 3):369–71. https://doi.org/10.1007/s00586-015-3929-7.
25. Wang MY, Mummaneni PV. Minimally invasive surgery for thoracolumbar spinal deformity: initial clinical experience with clinical and radiographic outcomes. Neurosurg Focus. 2010;28:E9. https://doi.org/10.3171/2010.1.focus09286.

Chapter 8
Oblique Lateral Lumbar Interbody Fusion: OLIF

Ronald Moskovich and Saqib Hasan

Introduction

Oblique lateral lumbar interbody fusion (OLIF) is a minimally invasive oblique lateral approach to the lumbar spine to perform interbody fusion. The dissection plane is extraperitoneal and provides access to the discs anterior to the psoas muscle [1, 2].

Ventral approaches for decompression and fusion of the lumbar spine to treat spinal tuberculosis were reported, in 1956, by A.R. Hodgeson and F.E. Stock [3]. Anterior approaches to the spine evolved to manage additional spinal conditions, including degenerative and deformity issues. However, there remained guarded enthusiasm, given the trepidation for violation of the abdominal or thoracic cavities, events traditionally associated with higher rates of morbidity and mortality. The development of structural interbody prostheses and modern spinal fixation devices played a significant role in enhancing reliability and safety, yet still necessitated significant open surgical exposure. OLIF represents a minimally invasive modification of the earlier anterior retroperitoneal flank approaches [4]. This technique also uniquely permits anterior access to L5-S1, which is not accessible using the lateral approach.

Indications

A plethora of literature exists supporting the use of interbody techniques for obtaining fusion for degenerative disc disease, degenerative scoliosis [5, 6], spondylolisthesis [7], spinal stenosis [8], adjacent segment disease [9], and recurrent disc herniation [10]. Experience with the OLIF is increasing with the variety of these conditions and appears positive [11].

R. Moskovich (✉) • S. Hasan
Department of Orthopedic Surgery, NYU Langone Health, New York, NY, USA
e-mail: Ronald.Moskovich@nyumc.org

G. Tender (ed.), *Minimally Invasive Spine Surgery Techniques*,
https://doi.org/10.1007/978-3-319-71943-6_8

Interbody fusion may, at present, be considered a reliable option for degenerative spondylolisthesis with pre-operative segmental instability and as a treatment for pseudarthrosis following posterolateral fusion [12]. Moreover, interbody techniques should be considered a critical part of the spine surgeon's armamentarium for addressing lumbar spine pathology to achieve high rates of fusion, depending on patient-specific factors and surgeon comfort with the technique.

Advantages for utilizing interbody fusion include:

- Biomechanical: Fusion close to the longitudinal bending axis of the spine and in line with the compression moments of the vertebral bodies enhances the load-bearing force through the fusion bed.
- Biological: The rich blood supply from the cancellous fusion bed is exposed. A larger graft placement further increases surface area to facilitate fusion.
- Decompression: Distraction of the disc space and neuroforamina results in indirect decompression.
- Spinal balance: Restoration of segmental lordosis and coronal realignment via appropriate placement of interbody grafts improves overall weight distribution and stability.

Alternative treatment options for interbody fusion include:

- Anterior lumbar interbody fusion
- Transforaminal lumbar interbody fusion
- Posterior lumbar interbody fusion
- Lateral lumbar interbody fusion

Evolution

The traditional anterior retroperitoneal approach is performed with the patient in a lateral oblique position. An oblique flank incision is made with wide dissection of the abdominal muscles. Extraperitoneal dissection, segmental vascular ligation, and mobilization of the aorta and inferior vena cava provide access to the anterior aspect of the lumbar spine (Fig. 8.1). Distal extension of this incision permits access over

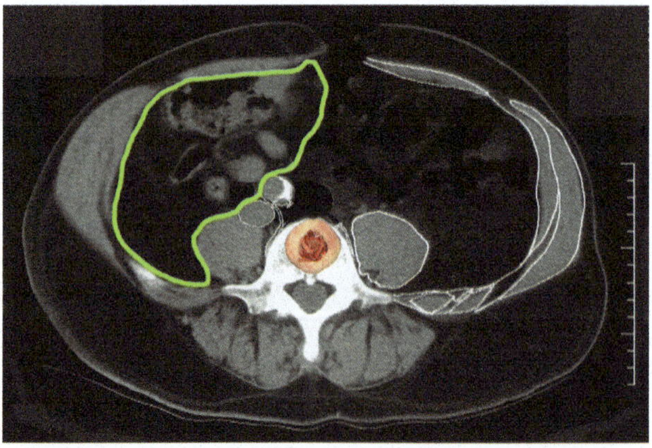

Fig. 8.1 Cross-sectional CT of the lumbar spine at L4–5, demonstrating the considerable degree of visceral retraction required for open anterior lumbar interbody fusion (ALIF)

the great vessels and iliac vessels to the L5–S1 interspace, if needed. This extensile exposure does necessitate segmental vascular control and mobilization to expose the intervertebral discs. We have often encountered prevertebral adhesions adjacent to a severely arthritic disc or at a spondylolisthetic level, possibly a response to local inflammatory reaction at the disc level. The great vessels and venous tributaries may have fibrous adhesions to the disc annulus, which complicates vascular mobilization and increases the risk of vascular injury, both during access and retraction [13]. Iliolumbar vein ligation and transection is necessary to permit medial retraction of the common iliac vein to ensure adequate anterior exposure of the L4–5 disc [14]. Postoperative abdominal wall paralysis or atony may be a complication of extended muscle wall dissection, and asymmetric abdominal wall distension may give the appearance of an abdominal hernia.

A variation of the above technique, with the patient in a supine position, uses an anterior incision medial to the rectus abdominis muscle that avoids injury to the oblique and transversus abdominis muscles and their segmental nerve supply. Use of this modification does not obviate the need for segmental vascular dissection and firm retraction of the great vessels. Because the patient is supine, active retraction of the peritoneum and its contents is necessary, as these structures do not passively fall away from the spine. Alternatively, anterior transperitoneal or extraperitoneal access to the lumbosacral disc may be used, with similar caveats regarding vascular dissection and visceral retraction (Fig. 8.2).

Lateral Interbody Fusion

Oval-shaped, large footprint interbody cages inserted through a lateral trans-psoas approach revolutionized the surgery of lumbar interbody arthrodesis. The extreme lateral interbody fusion (XLIF) and direct lateral interbody fusion (DLIF) permit less invasive access to the lumbar disc spaces [15–17]. The cages are designed to restore coronal and sagittal spinal alignment. These procedures, however, place the lumbar nerve roots and lumbar plexus at risk of injury, as they exit deep to and pass

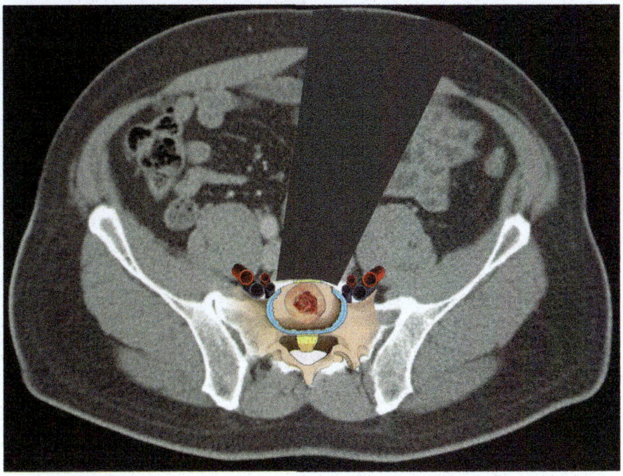

Fig. 8.2 Cross-sectional CT demonstrating the visceral retraction required to place a lumbar interbody graft at L5–S. The iliac vessels diverge bilaterally

through the substance of the psoas muscle. Intraoperative neurophysiologic monitoring using specialized probes and instruments is helpful to identify the nerves. Muscle relaxant use to ease surgical retraction may interfere with neurophysiologic monitoring.

For the XLIF procedure, patients are placed in a direct lateral decubitus position on the operating table and are usually laterally flexed or jack-knifed over the table break, which stretches and tensions the lumbar plexus. Surgery should be performed expeditiously to limit the time that the nerves are stretched. Jack-knife positioning for 60 min has been demonstrated to cause transient neuropraxia [18].

A similar extraperitoneal approach is used for OLIF; however, the extraperitoneal dissection continues anterior to the psoas muscle (ante-psoas), and similarly minimizes the visceral retraction needed. When performing the OLIF procedure, the patient is placed on a flat operating table in an anatomic position on his/her side with the legs straight so that the nerves are anatomically relaxed, which minimizes the necessity for neural monitoring, and large footprint interbody cages can be inserted (Fig. 8.3).

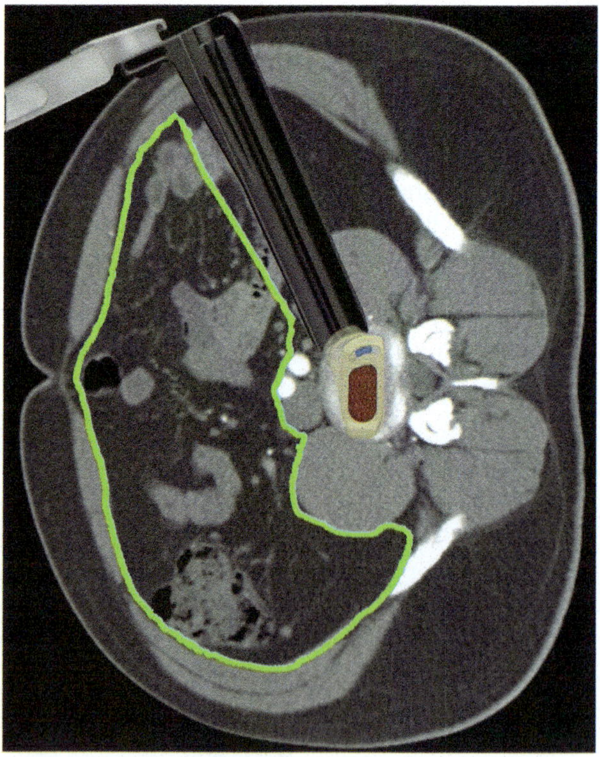

Fig. 8.3 Cross-sectional CT of the lumbar spine at the L4–5 level with the patient in the lateral decubitus position. Very little visceral retraction is required for the OLIF. The proximally placed radiolucent inserter is seen, with the interbody cage in position

Preoperative Evaluation

Patients with a history of previous retroperitoneal procedures may preclude use of this technique due to retroperitoneal scarring and adhesions. Prior intraperitoneal operations and laparoscopic procedures are usually not associated with peritoneal fibrosis and do not contraindicate OLIF surgery [19].

Patients with degenerative lumbar spinal pathology who are able to benefit from this technique may have clinical symptomatology related to:

- Loss of disc height with neuroforaminal stenosis
- Radicular pain associated with a component of axial pain
- Coronal or sagittal imbalance associated with scoliosis
- Segmental instability associated with moderate lateral olisthesis and grade 1–2 spondylolisthesis

Imaging

Radiographs

- Examination of overall alignment, degree of spondylosis, and segmental instability.
- Evaluation of the level of iliac crests, particularly, when accessing L4–5 disc space. This may effect placement of the incision.

Magnetic Resonance Imaging (MRI)

- MRI is used to evaluate neuroforamina and compression related to disc height collapse and spondylotic changes, resulting in dorsal compression from facet hypertrophy and mass effect from the ligamentum flavum, and to assess the need for direct decompression if indirect decompression is unlikely to address the type of stenosis present.
- MRI is also used to evaluate the morphology of the psoas musculature and the corridor between the vessels and the psoas muscle for access to the disc space. Additionally, a well visualized fat plane between the psoas muscle and the disc indicates that the psoas can be more easily retracted (Fig. 8.4). Aortic aneurysm or aortic tortuosity may contraindicate anterior surgery. This evaluation is critical to ascertain that an adequate corridor exists in order to minimize vessel trauma when accessing the disc space [20, 21].
- An anatomic study using MRI measured the corridor between the anterior border of the psoas muscle and the anterior great vessels from L2 to S1, revealed adequate working space with minimal psoas retraction [22] (Table 8.1).

Computed Tomography (CT) Myelography

- CT is useful in patients unable to be evaluated by MRI and may be better for osseous evaluation and previous placement of internal fixation.

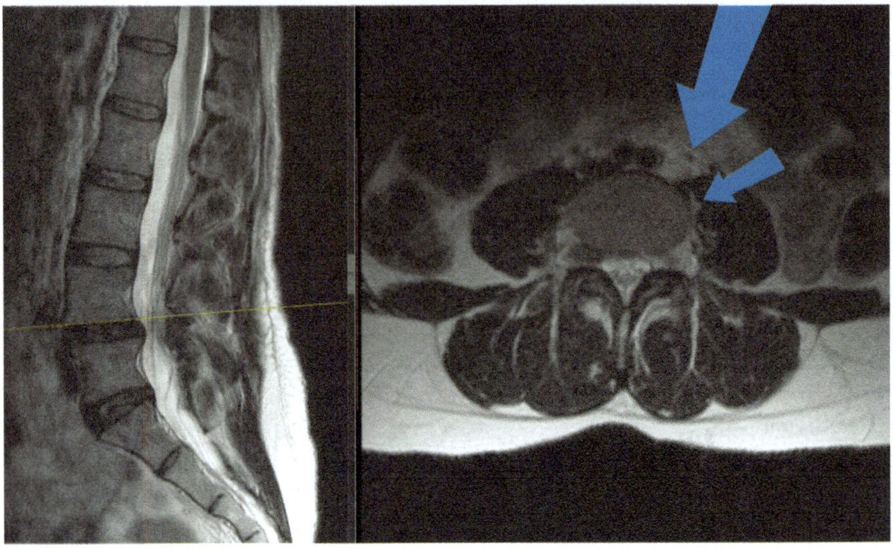

Fig. 8.4 Corridor between the vessels and the psoas muscle for access to the disc space—Large arrow. The fat plane between the psoas muscle and the disc at L4–5—Small arrow

Table 8.1 Corridor between the anterior border of the psoas muscles and the anterior great vessels from L2 to S1

Space	Unretracted psoas	Retracted psoas
L2–L3	18.0 mm	24.9 mm
L3–L4	18.8 mm	26.3 mm
L4–L5	14.4 mm	23.6 mm
L5–S1	15.2 mm	24.8 mm

Surgical Technique

Relevant Anatomy

Safe access to the anterior lumbar spine necessitates an intimate understanding of the segmental anatomy. Importantly, the cross sectional and longitudinal anatomy changes three-dimensionally from the thoracolumbar junction to the lumbosacral level. Knowledge of this anatomy is essential when performing OLIF approaches.

The L2–3, L3–4 and L4–5 discs are generally accessible; hence, the OLIF25 moniker for these procedures. Access to L1–2 may be possible, as the eleventh and twelfth ribs are "floating ribs" that are not attached to the sternum, so that the surgeon is able to retract and displace them. Due to the dome-shaped diaphragm, the pulmonary cavity extends distal to the diaphragmatic apex. A skin incision distal to the twelfth rib will generally avoid entering the costophrenic recess of the pleural cavity, which would result in a pneumothorax.

The sympathetic chain generally lies medial to the psoas muscle and can be mobilized further anteriorly with blunt dissection using a Kittner. Direct lateral

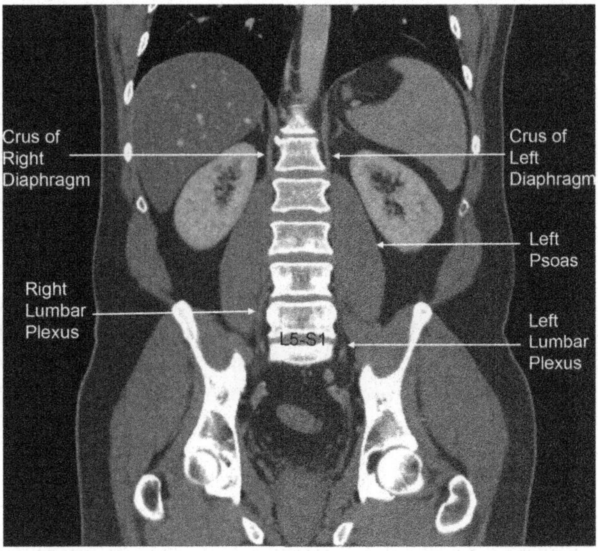

Fig. 8.5 CT demonstrating the lower lumbar plexus in the coronal plane. The crura of the diaphragm, the liver on the right, spleen on the left, and kidneys are visualized

exposures of the lumbar spine endanger the lumbar nerve roots, which exit the spine via the intervertebral foramina and generally lie deep to or within the psoas major muscles, where they form the lumbar plexus (Fig. 8.5). The iliohypogastric and ilioinguinal nerves (which arise from the first lumbar nerve and a twig from T12) pass through the posterior border of the psoas major, and lie anterior to the fascia over the psoas muscle. They may be somewhat bound to the muscle by the medial continuation of the transversalis fascia, where they are at risk of injury from direct lateral access. The genitofemoral nerve is also at risk as it arises from the first and second lumbar roots, pierces the psoas major and runs near its anterior border. Dissection anterior to the psoas major rather than through the muscle (trans-psoas) reduces the potential to injure the lumbar plexus. The motor nerves are generally located in the posterior third of the psoas major but may be located more anteriorly in the lower lumbar levels [23]. The femoral nerve is at particular risk at L4–5. These nerves are also endangered from prolonged psoas retraction.

The ureter runs anteromedial to the psoas muscle and is usually mobilized with the peritoneum. Also, descending in the extraperitoneal space are gonadal vessels. The testicular artery in males and the ovarian artery in females may be identified on preoperative axial MRI and are often visualized intraoperatively. These structures should be mobilized anteriorly. A segmental artery and vein originate from the aorta and vena cava at the level of the middle of each lumbar vertebra from L1 to L5 and can be identified at each level by their position and horizontal lie.

Access from the left side is generally preferred considering the more robust aortic vessel wall, compared to the right-sided vena cava, and the usually wider corridor between the aorta and the psoas on the left side, compared to that between the vena cava and the psoas. When utilizing the OLIF approach, mobilization of the retroperitoneal structures anteriorly and towards the dependent, opposite side, provides adequate access to the lateral aspect of the discs and does not usually require vascular division. Care should be taken with placement of lateral positioning pins within the vertebral body to avoid the segmental artery. If necessary, one or more segmental vessels may be ligated and divided. The use of an arthroscopic knot pusher facilitates safe knot tying through the small external apertures.

The abdominal aorta divides at about the fourth lumbar vertebra into the right and left common iliac arteries. These arteries descend anteromedial to the L5 vertebra and lumbosacral disc. The iliolumbar vein, or ascending lumbar vein, arises variably from the proximal common iliac vein and usually requires ligation in order to safely mobilize the common iliac vessels medially when performing an anterior approach to the disc [24]. The vessel may be branched or may have a dual origin from the vessel, further complicating ligation and mobilization. The OLIF approach usually obviates the need for ligation of these vessels; however, direct visualization to assure that they are not in the operative field is essential. The sympathetic nerves may be visualized and also mobilized anteriorly to assist exposure of the lateral aspect of the intervertebral disc.

Equipment

- Flat radiolucent table
- Fluoroscopic imaging
- 3D Navigation (optional)
- Specialized minimally-invasive retractors
- Microscope or endoscope (when performing direct decompression)

Positioning

The patient is placed in the right lateral decubitus position on a flat radiolucent operating table and close to the front of the table, as the primary surgeon operates while standing anteriorly to the patient. An advantage of the more anterior patient positioning is that the abdomen falls away from the operative side and may even extend over the anterior edge of the operating table, providing advantage to the surgeon having to deal with the anterior adiposity.

An axillary roll should be used to protect the brachial plexus. The arms should be placed almost perpendicular to the thorax and supported on vertically parallel arm boards. The patient's trunk is stabilized with adhesive tape wrapped over the thorax and pelvis and affixed directly to the table. A small folded towel under the inferior rib cage and possibly the flank often help realign the lumbar spine.

The spine should be assessed fluoroscopically during positioning to ensure true perpendicular alignment to the operating table, so that an orthogonal lateral approach to the discs and implant insertion and its position can be monitored (Fig. 8.6). A pillow should be placed between the legs to maintain a neutral alignment of the pelvis perpendicular to the spine with the legs in a relatively straight position.

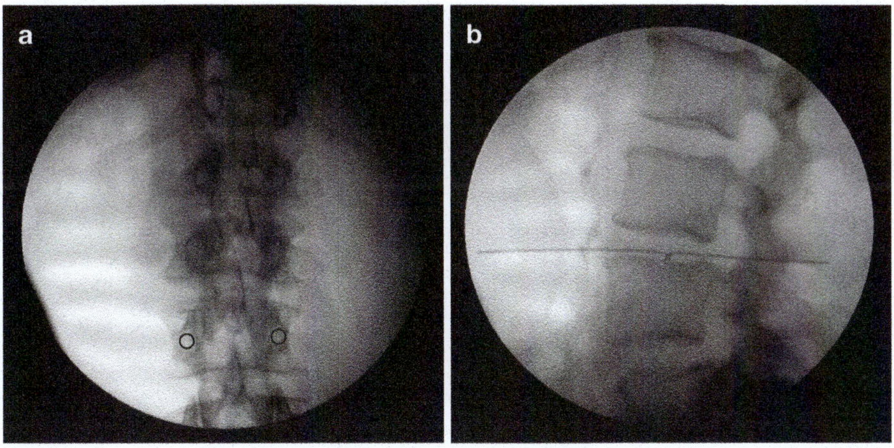

Fig. 8.6 Fluoroscopic anteroposterior view of the symmetric L3 pedicles (outlined), spinous processes in the midline, and a true lateral of the lumbar spine confirms perpendicular alignment of the spine to the operating table. The lateral radiographic marker identifies the anteroposterior midline of the L3–4 disc

The neutral, straight position of the legs relaxes the psoas muscle and minimizes trauma during its retraction.

The fluoroscope C-arm is covered with sterile drapes so that both anteroposterior and lateral views of the spine may be obtained. Additionally, computerized image guidance using appropriate tools may be utilized.

Neuromonitoring is not essential for OLIF surgery but may be deployed at the surgeon's preference. Establishing baseline neurophysiological measurements prior to skin incision may be performed to compare with those obtained if subsequent posterior internal fixation is anticipated.

OLIF25

Skin Marking

The iliac crest position is marked on the skin. Radiopaque markers are used to identify the anterior and posterior margins of the vertebral bodies and the discs, which are then drawn on the skin using a pen. The direction or obliquity of the intervertebral disc spaces is also marked and the midline of vertebral bodies identified. The line drawn over the disc is extended anteriorly 5 cm to indicate the planned incision. If the L4–5 level is to be accessed and that level is associated with a relatively high iliac crest, the line of the disc should be extended a further 2 cm anteriorly to take advantage of the lower position of the anterior iliac crest. The skin incision may be horizontal for one-level access but a short vertical incision is generally used, as it may provide a somewhat more extensile access. If two levels are exposed, the incision may be made between the two levels and the skin gently mobilized up and down (Figs. 8.7 and 8.8).

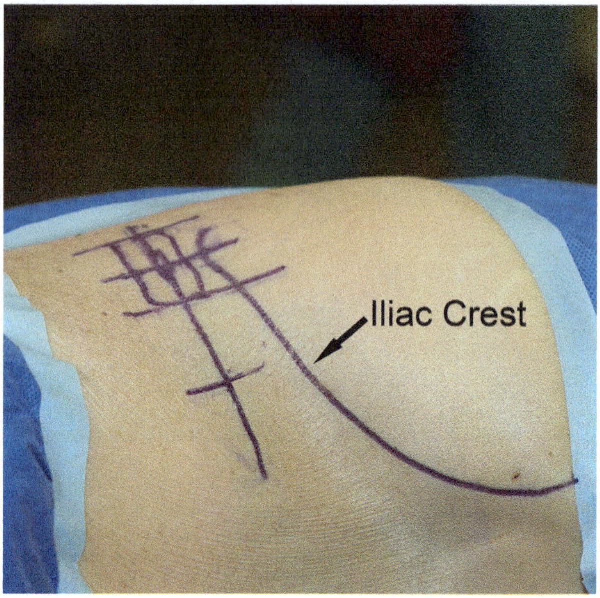

Fig. 8.7 Skin marking of the L3–4 disc space, based on the fluoroscopic images. The midline of the disc is projected anteriorly approximately 5 cm to indicate the skin incision

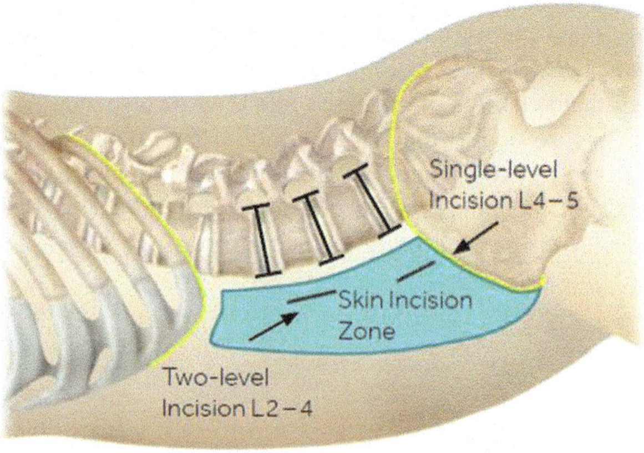

Fig. 8.8 Diagram of the skin incision zones

Superficial Dissection

The dissection is continued through the subcutaneous tissue to the external oblique muscle. The external oblique fibers are separated using a hemostat, small scissors, or a dissecting sponge. The internal oblique muscle is then similarly split, almost perpendicular to the external oblique. The horizontally aligned transversus abdominis muscle is exposed and split along the line of its fibers. Transection of the muscle fibers themselves is not necessary, as in the old McBurney grid-iron appendicectomy exposure.

Deep Surgical Dissection

The peritoneum is usually visualized immediately deep to the transversus abdominis muscles. The surgeon's index finger is introduced and directed horizontally and posteriorly to sweep the peritoneum off the posterior lateral abdominal wall (Fig. 8.9). If the peritoneum is penetrated or incised, a surrounding area of peritoneum should be exposed and repaired with a suture. The peritoneum is further mobilized off the posterior abdominal wall, extending down to the psoas muscle where the peritoneum is similarly progressively mobilized anteriorly over the psoas muscle.

As soon as the extraperitoneal space is entered, a small handheld retractor with fiberoptic lighting may be introduced and further dissection performed under direct vision. The ilio-inguinal, ilio-hypogastric, and genitofemoral nerves and the ureter

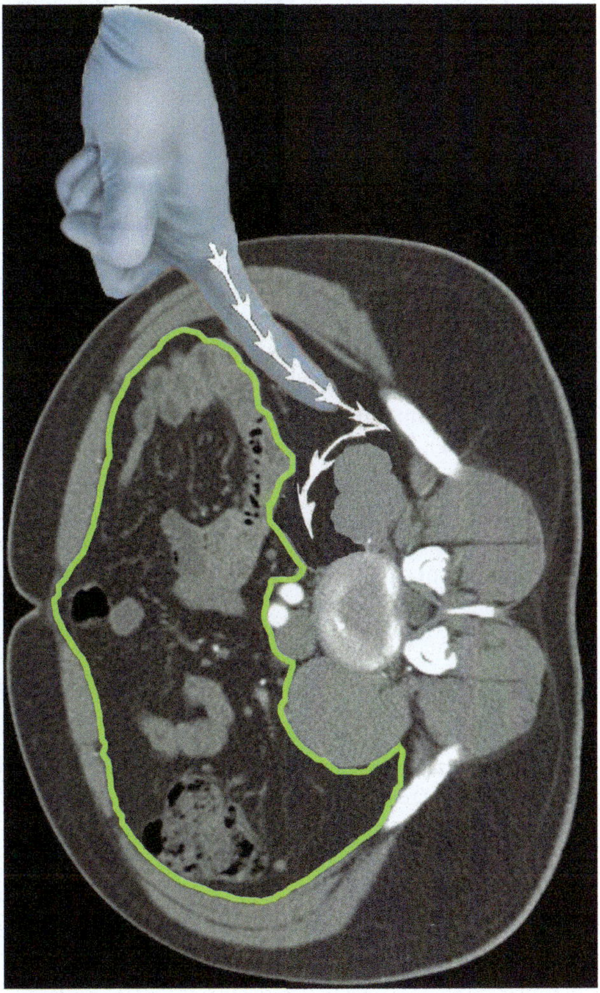

Fig. 8.9 Trajectory of the extraperitoneal dissection. The peritoneum (yellow) is separated from the posterior lateral abdominal wall, then down and anterior to the psoas muscle

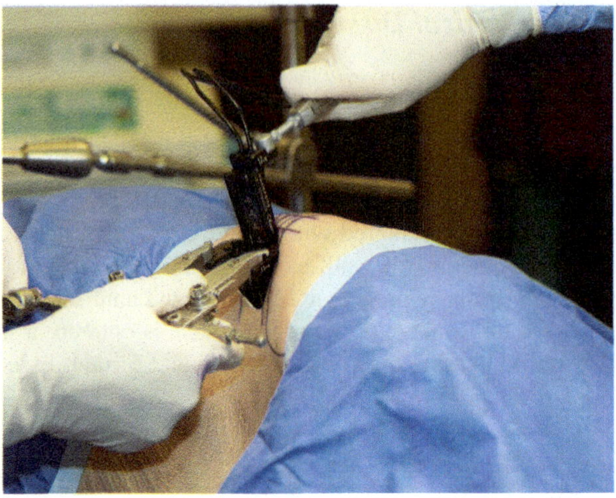

Fig. 8.10 The handheld, fiberoptically illuminated retractor is used to assist dissection and to gauge the depth of the incision. Self-retaining retractors of appropriate blade length are then inserted

are mobilized anteriorly. The psoas muscle is, thus, progressively denuded of soft tissue. It is important to ensure that the peritoneum is completely mobilized anteriorly and a direct view of the naked psoas muscle is obtained. The anterior border of the psoas muscle may then be retracted posteriorly over a short distance. Kittner sponges or a Cobb elevator may be utilized to mobilize the muscle and expose the lateral aspect of the disc. Anteroposterior and lateral radiographic confirmation of position is obtained.

Radiolucent blade retractors can be introduced. These should be placed above and below the intervertebral disc being operated (Fig. 8.10). Retractors affixed directly to the operating table are recommended as intraoperative radiography is used to control instrument positioning, making the use of handheld retractors difficult (Fig. 8.11). The retractor arms are spread to expose the width and depth of the lateral aspect of the disc. A retractor blade retaining pin may be inserted into the vertebra, close to the end plate to avoid damage to the segmental vessel. As the retractor is stabilized by its attachment to the table, only one pin is usually required, although pins may be placed in both the upper and lower blades.

Annulotomy, Discectomy, and Endplate Preparation

The direct lateral midline of the disc is confirmed radiographically. A rectangular annulotomy is created with an extended offset bayonet scalpel. A standard discectomy is then performed using Cobb elevators, curettes, and pituitary rongeurs. It is important to maintain an orthogonal line of access to the disc. Inadvertent dissection through the anterior annulus may result in vascular and neurological damage and posteriorly may compromise the nerve roots. Additionally, it may decrease the mechanical integrity of the anterior and posterior annulus fibrosus. The discectomy

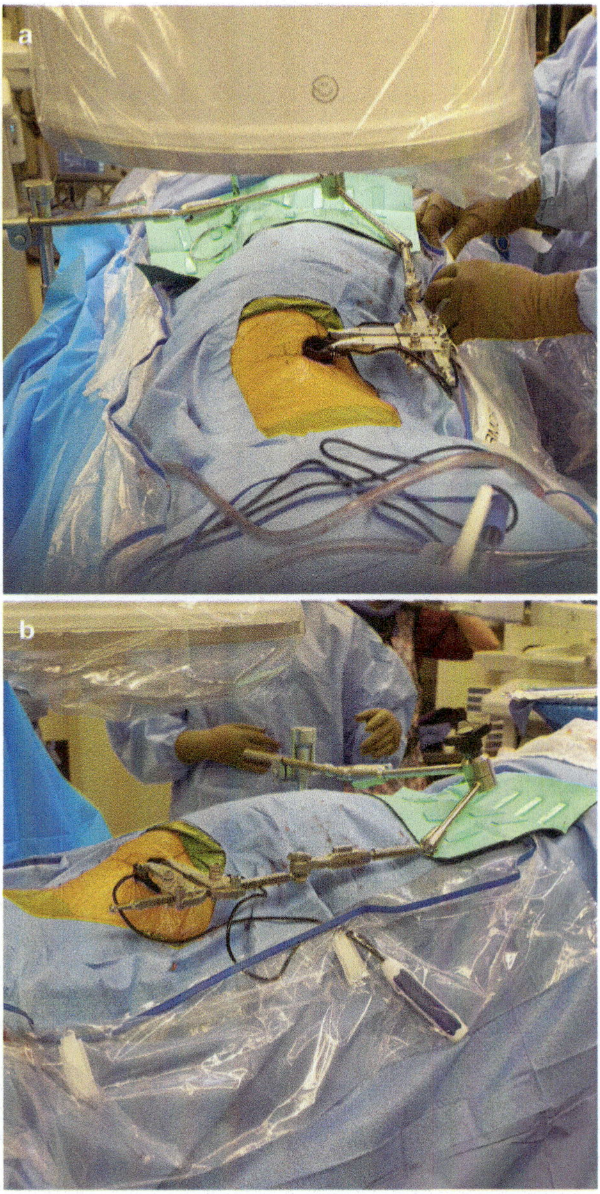

Fig. 8.11 (**a**) The self-retaining retractor blades are attached to the table-mounted armature, which is low profile and facilitates surgical access and radiographic control. View from the head of the patient. The patient's left-side is up. (**b**) View of the retractor placement from the front of the patient. The patient's head is to the left

is performed under direct vision or indirectly with fluoroscopic or image-guided control. The endplates are cleared of all soft tissue. An operating microscope may be introduced, if necessary, to further visualize the disc space or if a disc herniation or osteophyte resection is required.

Following completion of the discectomy, an elongated Cobb elevator is inserted and directed down over the upper and lower endplates of the disc space. Gentle mallet

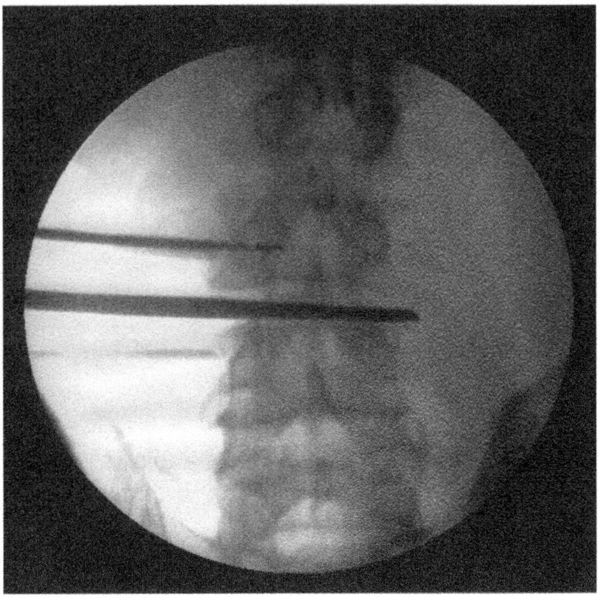

Fig. 8.12 The Cobb elevator is passed along the superior and inferior end plates to penetrate the opposite annulus following discectomy

blows on the Cobb elevator is utilized to penetrate and release the contralateral disc annulus. Fluoroscopic or image guidance is necessary (Fig. 8.12). The Cobb elevator should just penetrate the contralateral annulus on both the up and down side surfaces of the intervertebral space. Care should be taken not to penetrate more than a few millimeters through the opposite side to avoid the risk of injury to the plexus or precipitate a hematoma in the contralateral psoas muscle [25]. Intervertebral metal trial prostheses are then utilized to assess the intervertebral dimensions and select an appropriate sized interbody cage.

Note that the anterior longitudinal ligament can be visualized utilizing this approach and may be released for deformity correction as needed [26]. This is unnecessary in most cases, and carries the risk of compromising the anterior soft tissue envelope of the disc space, as well as risk of vascular injury. Similarly, care should be taken not to violate the posterior annulus [27].

Implant Trialing and Final Implant Insertion

Emphasis is again placed on the establishment of an orthogonal position of the implant. The lateral width and anteroposterior size of the disc space is evaluated by inserting trial prostheses to assess anteroposterior dimension, width of the vertebra, interbody height, and lordosis (Figs. 8.13 and 8.14). An appropriate lumbar cage is then selected and the cage is filled with bone allograft or material of the surgeon's choice. Our preference is to use a cage with integrated directional locking flanges or other surface treatment that resists back-out of the cage following insertion

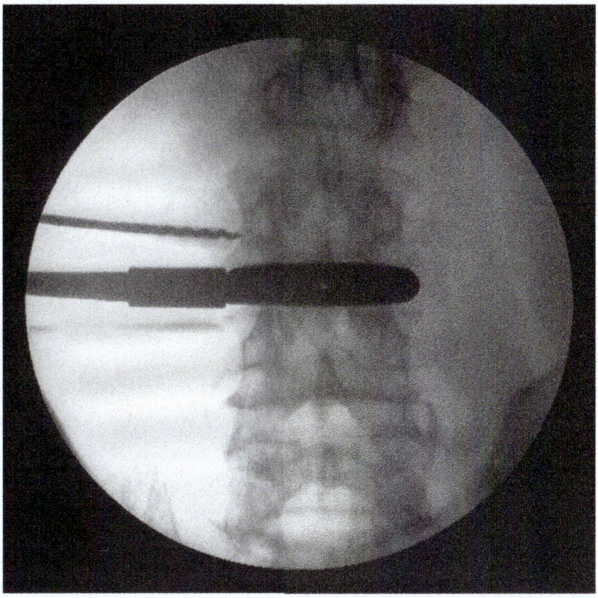

Fig. 8.13 The trial prosthesis is inserted. The radiographic "bulls-eye" at the midline helps confirm orthogonal trial placement. Biplane radiographic confirmation should be elicited to assess graft height, width, and depth. Prosthesis selection depends on accurate templating

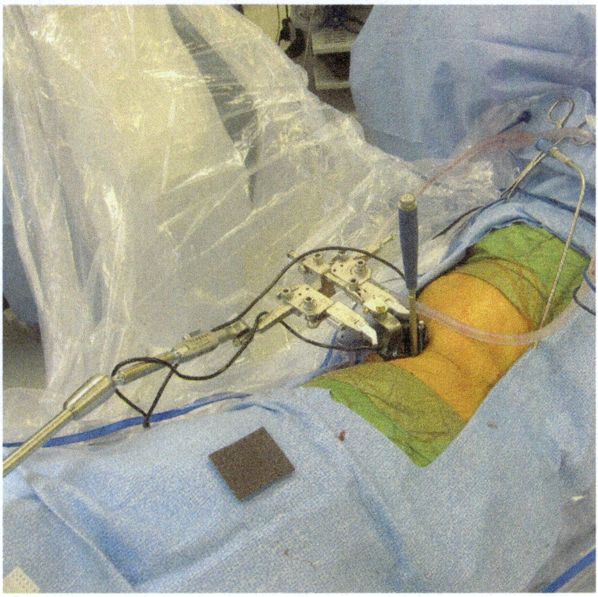

Fig. 8.14 AP radiographic set-up. The trial prosthesis insertion handle is perpendicular to the spine, which adds confirmation of orthogonal placement

(Fig. 8.15). For this reason, it is also important to ensure that the correct size prosthesis is selected. Reposition or removal of a prosthesis with other than a relatively smooth surface may result in damage to the vertebral endplates, as the surface may act like a rasp during prosthesis removal.

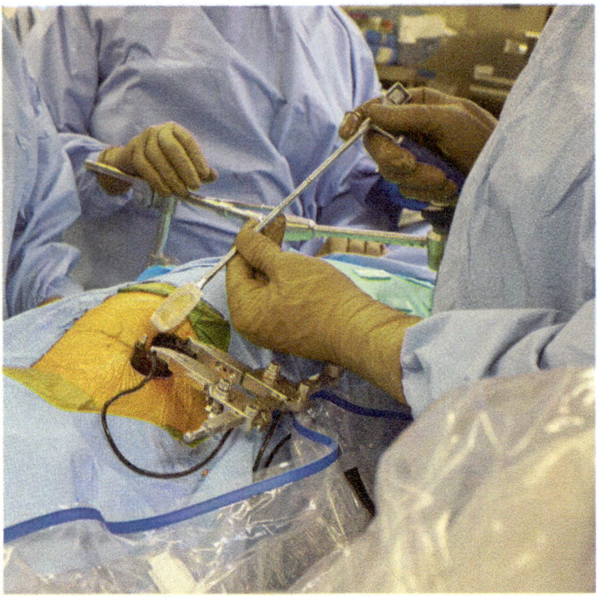

Fig. 8.15 The interbody prosthesis affixed to the inserter prior to implantation

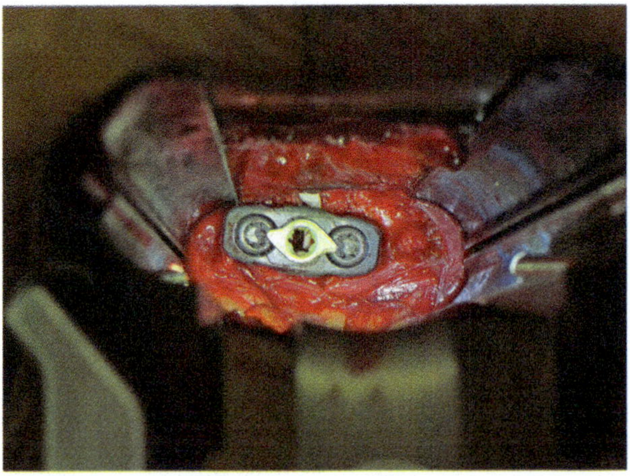

Fig. 8.16 Lateral lumbar plate backing up the interbody arthrodesis

Following insertion of the cage, a lateral plate can be deployed if necessary (Fig. 8.16). The retractor retaining pin(s) should be removed. A small amount of bone wax may be impressed into the retaining pinhole(s) for hemostasis.

Clinical cases: Figs. 8.17, 8.18 and 8.19

Multi-Level Fusion

Following insertion of the prosthesis and completion of the OLIF, the retractors may be repositioned at the adjacent level, if indicated, and a discectomy and interbody cage placement performed utilizing the above described technique. The self-retaining

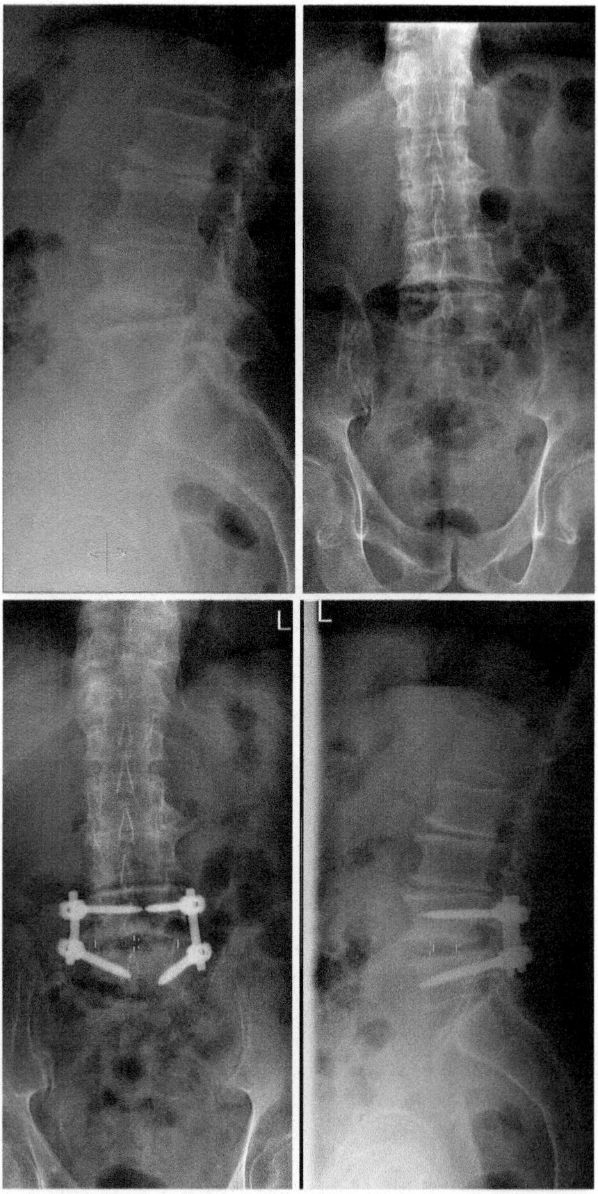

Fig. 8.17 (**a**) Standing lateral and AP radiographs of a 72-year-old man with marked lumbar stenosis and predominantly right radiculopathy. Note the asymmetric coronal disc narrowing at L4–5. (**b**) Three-month postoperative radiographs following OLIF at L4–5 and minimally invasive pedicle screw fixation. The patient experienced an early return to activity and achieved full function with neurologic recovery. He remained well, and radiographs taken a year postoperatively showed further maturation of the fusion

retractors may then be removed. Direct visualization of the removal tract is helpful to monitor integrity of the peritoneum and the anatomic structures displaced during the procedure. Hemostasis should also be confirmed. Separate closure of each of the three muscle layers is done, followed by subcutaneous and subcuticular skin closure.

For a two- or three-level fusion, the skin may be mobilized proximally or distally, and separate transmuscular dissections performed through the three abdominal wall muscle layers, rather than extending the primary intermuscular dissection. This technique minimizes dissection and retraction, as less extensile muscle dissection is required.

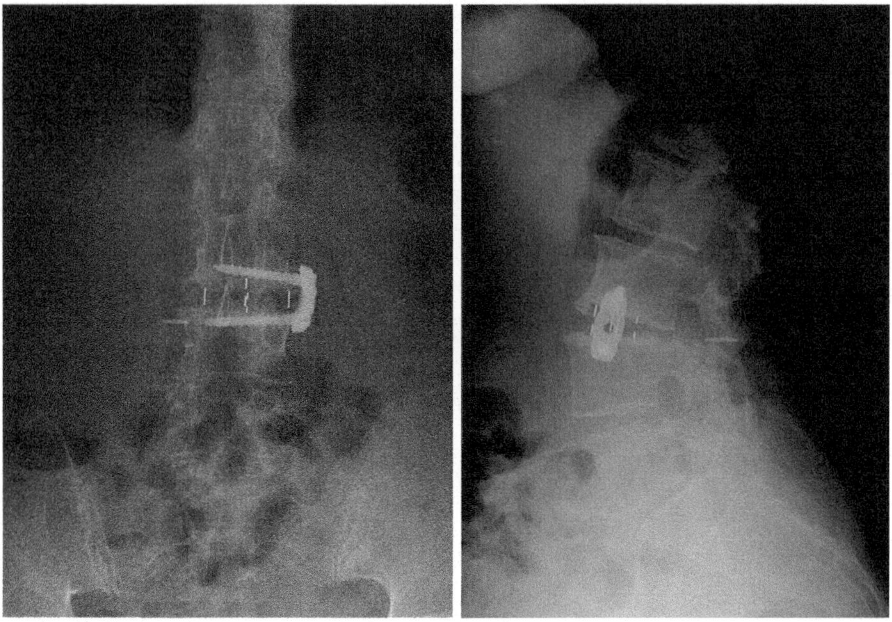

Fig. 8.18 Standing AP and lateral radiographs of a 66-year-old patient who developed spinal stenosis adjacent to an old L4–5 fusion. A stand-alone L3–4 OLIF was performed with a lateral plate for supplemental anterior fixation. An intraoperative view of the plate is documented in Fig. 8.16

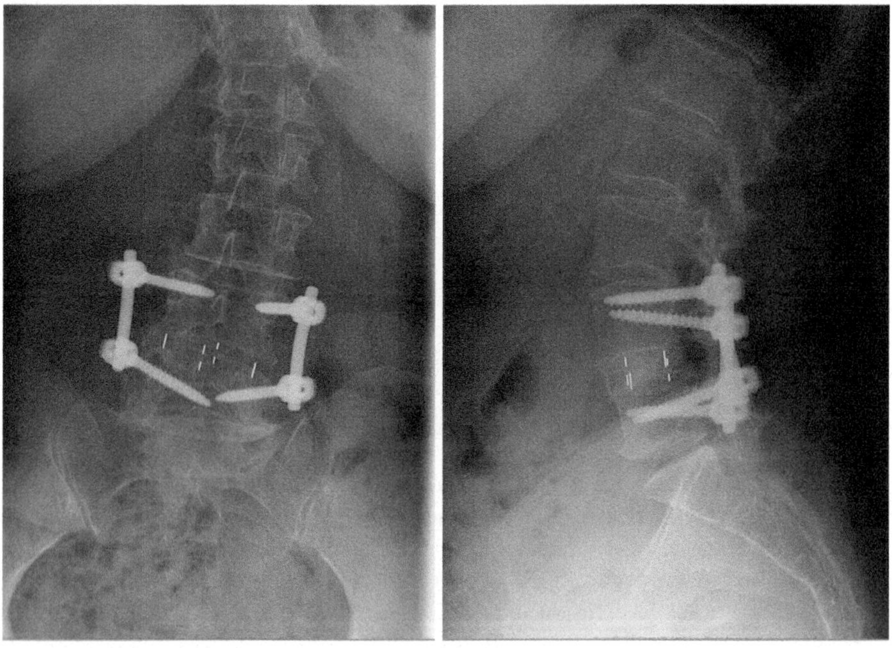

Fig. 8.19 Radiographs 11 months following OLIF and pedicle screw arthrodesis to treat L4–5 spondylolisthesis and stenosis in a 65 year old who also had mild scoliosis. The patient had a good clinical outcome. Bone growth through and anterior to the prosthesis is visible

OLIF51

Oblique lateral interbody fusion at L5–S1 (OLIF51) is also possible in the lateral position, as a stand-alone procedure or in addition to proximal-level arthrodesis using an extension of the OLIF25 incision. A modification of the OLIF25 technique is utilized. The location of the anterior iliac crest is marked on the skin. The L5–S1 intervertebral disc is identified fluoroscopically using a metal skin marker. A line is drawn over the center of the disc and projected forward to identify the slope and the lordosis of the L5-S1 disc space. A second line is drawn from the center of the disc extending anteriorly and perpendicular to the operating table as it is drawn onto the abdomen. This line represents the actual level of the disc in the abdomen and also marks the most cephalad border for the incision. A vertical line is then drawn about two fingerbreadths anterior to the anterior superior iliac spine. This connecting line identifies the line of the incision (Fig. 8.20).

The external oblique and internal oblique fibers are split in a similar manner to the technique described for OLIF25. At the L5–S1 level, the transversus abdominis muscle may be more of a light fascial structure. Extraperitoneal dissection is performed similarly to that described above. The dissection is continued anterior to the psoas muscle to expose the lower part of the great vessels and the common iliac vein and artery. The peritoneum is elevated over these vessels to expose the L5–S1 disc. This route provides direct access to the lumbosacral disc, albeit from a slightly oblique approach.

A fiberoptically illuminated radiolucent retractor, color coded green, is introduced and placed between the L5–S1 disc space and the right common iliac vessels, which it protects. A second retractor blade, color coded blue, is inserted to retract and protect the left common iliac vessels. A third retractor may be introduced to gently retract the vascular bifurcation proximally (Fig. 8.21). Using this set of

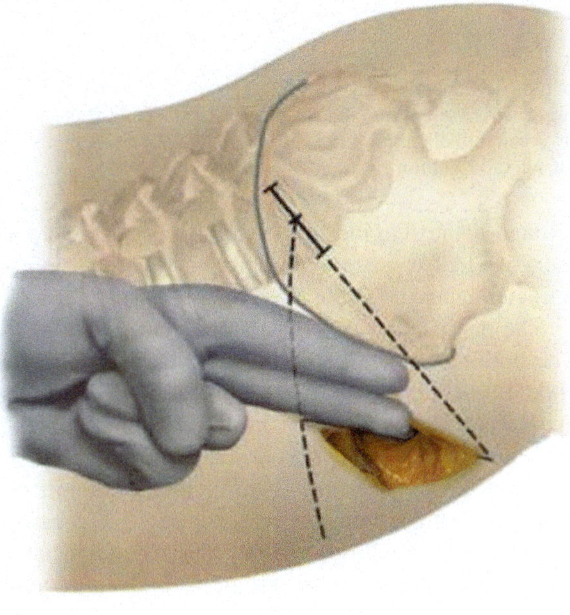

Fig. 8.20 Skin marking and incision for OLIF51 (See text)

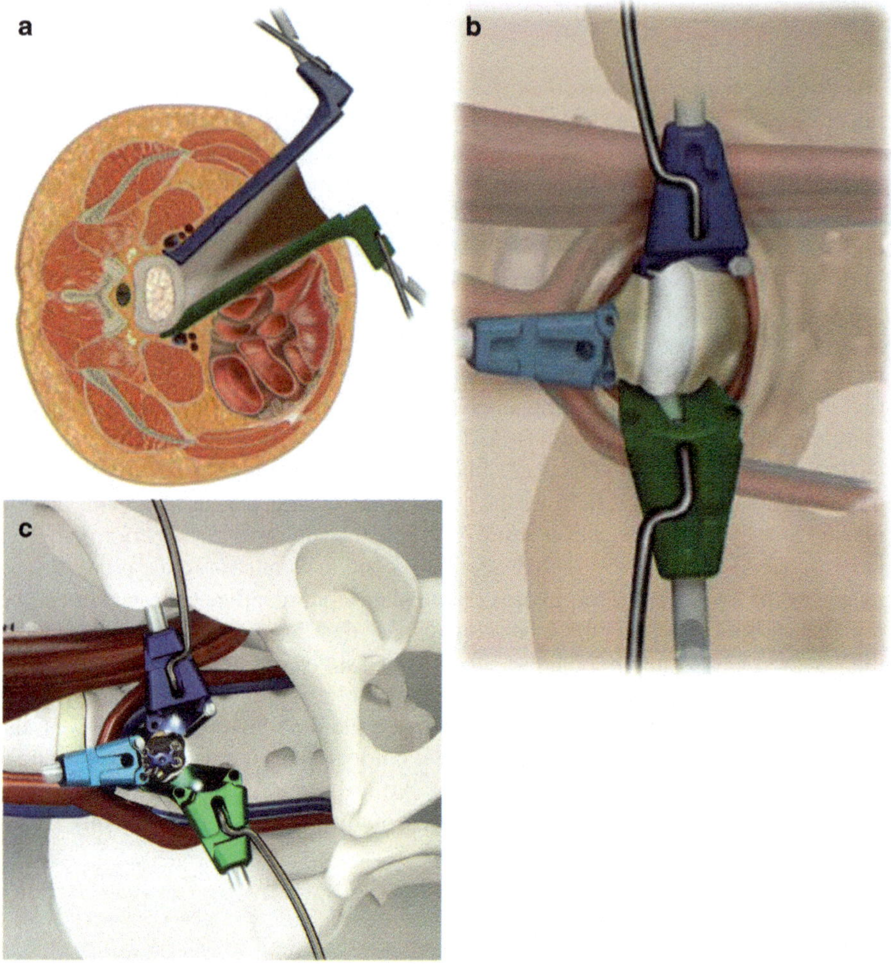

Fig. 8.21 (**a**) Superior and inferior OLIF51 retractor placement. (**b**) Proximal vascular retractor. (**c**) Anatomic diagram of the "anterior" OLIF51 retraction system and implant with the patient in the lateral decubitus position

retractors, the skin incision is mobilized somewhat more anterior and aligned with the L5–S1 disc space. A retaining screw may be passed through the blade of the retractor and fixed to the S1 vertebra (Fig. 8.22).

The median sacral vessels are visualized as they cross the midline of the disc. The midline is identified radiographically and marked. The median sacral vessels should be clipped or ligated and then divided. The superior hypogastric plexus are autonomic nerves situated on the vertebral bodies below the bifurcation of the abdominal aorta. These nerves should be mobilized away from the midline over the L5–S1 disc using a Kittner. This method of mobilization, rather than electrocautery transection, may diminish the incidence of retrograde ejaculation in males.

The L5–S1 annulus is incised anteriorly. An incision just to the left of midline may be helpful, as the approach is slightly oblique. A complete anterior discectomy is per-

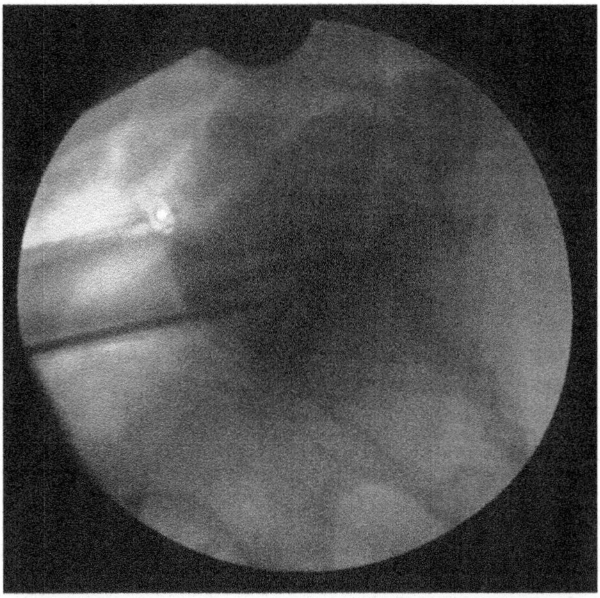

Fig. 8.22 Lateral view of the retaining screw passing through the retractor blade to the S1 vertebra

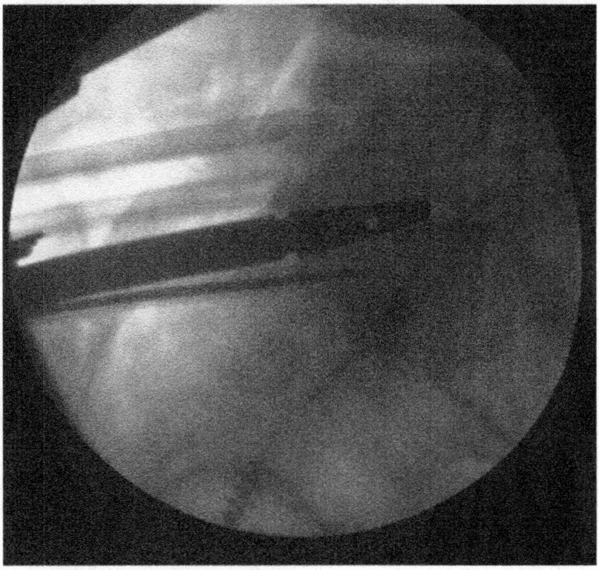

Fig. 8.23 Lateral view of the lordotic trial L5–S1 prosthesis in the correct orthogonal position

formed in the usual manner. The endplates of the vertebra are exposed. A trial prosthesis is selected. An off-set or straight-on insertion handle is used to accommodate the moderately oblique approach, yet maintain orthogonal position of the trial and the prosthesis. The trial is inserted into the intervertebral disc space. Orthogonal positioning of the trial is confirmed radiographically with reference to the bulls-eye viewed on the lateral radiograph (Fig. 8.23). Additional anteroposterior views may also be taken after temporary removal of the insertion rod. An appropriate interbody cage is selected

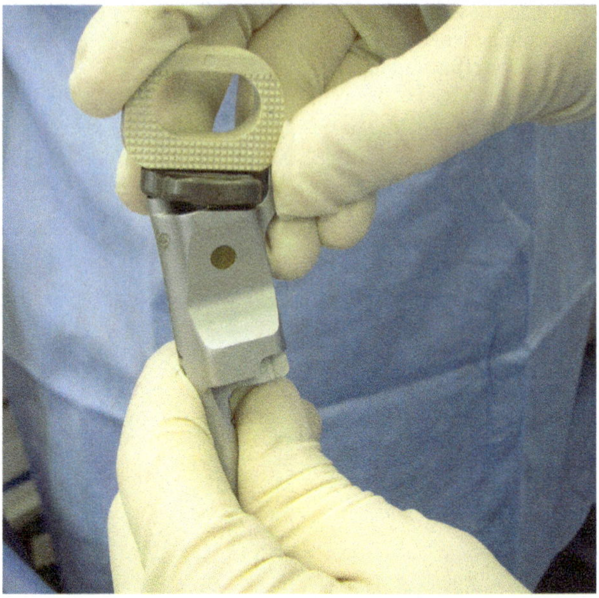

Fig. 8.24 PEEK L5–S1 interbody cage and retaining plate attached to an insertion rod

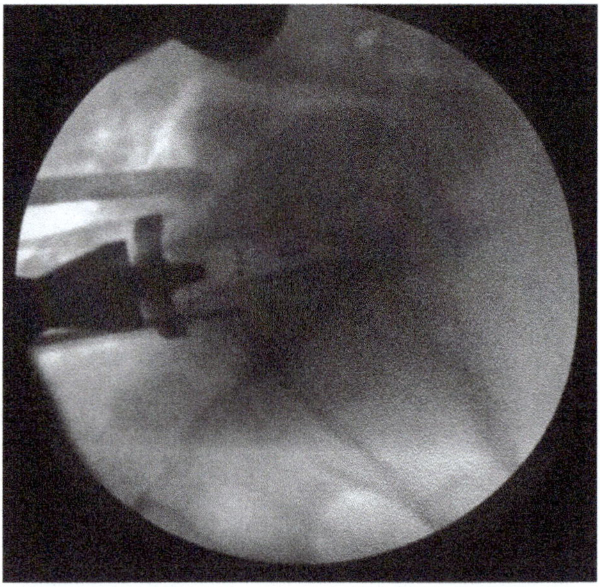

Fig. 8.25 Lateral view of the interbody cage and plate insertion. The metal markers indicate orthogonal position of the prosthesis

and attached to the insertion device. The choice of graft or prosthesis and the type of anterior fixation will vary depending on surgeon preference. In the example demonstrated, the drill guide is integral with the insertion guide to aid in screw positioning. The anterior fixation plate may be included to be inserted simultaneously with the cage (Fig. 8.24). The wire markers built into the prosthesis can be visualized fluoroscopically to confirm correct positioning (Fig. 8.25). The inserter is removed follow-

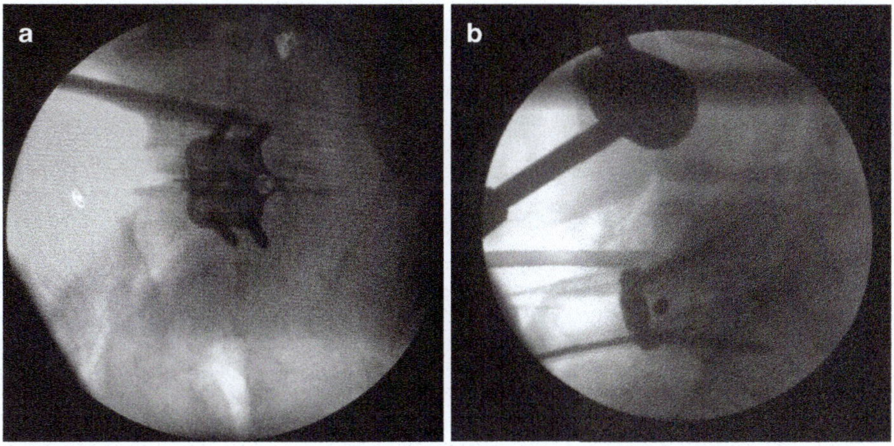

Fig. 8.26 (**a**) Radiographs demonstrating final implant position: (**a**) AP. (**b**) Lateral

Fig. 8.27 The L5–S1 plate screw-retaining flange has been deployed to prevent back-out. The left-sided (color coded blue) retractor blade is superior, the right-sided (color coded green) is inferior, and the superior vascular retractor is seen on the left side of this view. See also Fig. 8.21. The integral fiberoptic lighting illuminates the deep surgical field

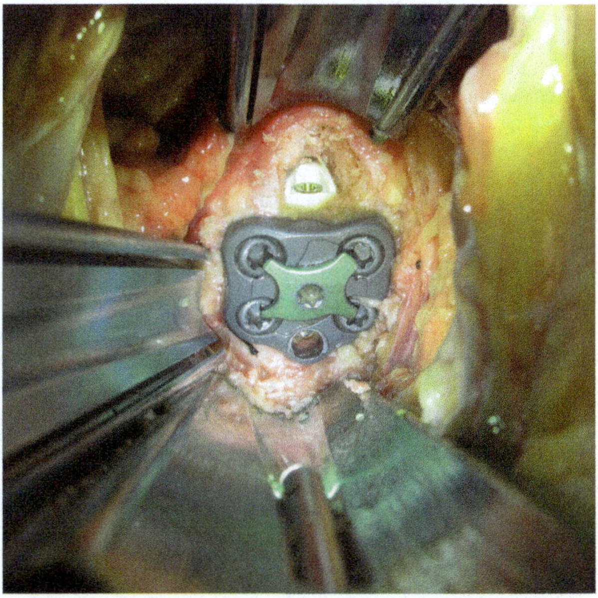

ing screw fixation of the plate and the screw retaining flange is deployed to prevent back-out (Figs. 8.26 and 8.27) The retroperitoneal space is examined as the retractors are removed under direct visualization. Muscle closure is performed in layers, followed by skin closure. During closure the iliohypogastric and ilioinguinal nerves should not be captured by the sutures.

Following completion of the anterior surgery, posterior fixation may be used at the surgeon's discretion. The stand-alone L5–S1 arthrodesis signals completion of the anterior surgery. The L5–S1 arthrodesis may be performed as a solitary procedure or combined with L4–5 or additional proximal levels, using the OLIF25 procedure described above.

References

1. Molloy S, Butler JS, Benton A, Malhotra K, Selvadurai S, Agu O. A new extensile anterolateral retroperitoneal approach for lumbar interbody fusion from L1 to S1: a prospective series with clinical outcomes. Spine J. 2016;16(6):786–91.
2. Woods KR, Billys JB, Hynes RA. Technical description of oblique lateral interbody fusion at L1-L5 (OLIF25) and at L5-S1 (OLIF51) and evaluation of complication and fusion rates. Spine J. 2017;17(4):545–53.
3. Hodgson AR, Stock FE. Anterior spinal fusion: A preliminary communication on the radical treatment of Pott's disease and Pott's paraplegia. Br. J. Surg. XLIV:266, 1956. Reprinted in Clin Orthop Relat Res. 1994 Mar;300:16-23 and 2006 Mar;444:10–5.
4. Mayer HM. A new microsurgical technique for minimally invasive anterior lumbar interbody fusion. Spine. 1997;22(6):691–9. discussion 700.
5. Anand N, Baron EM, Khandehroo B, Kahwaty S. Long-term 2- to 5-year clinical and functional outcomes of minimally invasive surgery for adult scoliosis. Spine. 2013;38(18):1566–75.
6. Phillips FM, Isaacs RE, Rodgers WB, Khajavi K, Tohmeh AG, Deviren V, et al. Adult degenerative scoliosis treated with XLIF: clinical and radiographical results of a prospective multicenter study with 24-month follow-up. Spine. 2013;38(21):1853–61.
7. Khajavi K, Shen A, Hutchison A. Substantial clinical benefit of minimally invasive lateral interbody fusion for degenerative spondylolisthesis. Eur Spine J. 2015;24(Suppl 3):314–21.
8. Castellvi AE, Nienke TW, Marulanda GA, Murtagh RD, Santoni BG. Indirect decompression of lumbar stenosis with transpsoas interbody cages and percutaneous posterior instrumentation. Clin Orthop Relat Res. 2014;472(6):1784–91.
9. Wang MY, Vasudevan R, Mindea SA. Minimally invasive lateral interbody fusion for the treatment of rostral adjacent-segment lumbar degenerative stenosis without supplemental pedicle screw fixation. J Neurosurg Spine. 2014;21(6):861–6.
10. Mroz TE, Lubelski D, Williams SK, O'Rourke C, Obuchowski NA, Wang JC, et al. Differences in the surgical treatment of recurrent lumbar disc herniation among spine surgeons in the United States. Spine J. 2014;14(10):2334–43.
11. Mehren C, Korge A. Minimally invasive anterior oblique lumbar interbody fusion (OLIF). Eur Spine J. 2016;25(Suppl 4):471–2.
12. Schroeder GD, Kepler CK, Kurd MF, Vaccaro AR, Hsu WK, Patel AA, et al. Rationale for the surgical treatment of lumbar degenerative spondylolisthesis. Spine. 2015;40(21):E1161–6.
13. Baker JK, Reardon PR, Reardon MJ, Heggeness MH. Vascular injury in anterior lumbar surgery. Spine. 1993;18(15):2227–30.
14. Unruh KP, Camp CL, Zietlow SP, Huddleston PM 3rd. Anatomical variations of the iliolumbar vein with application to the anterior retroperitoneal approach to the lumbar spine: a cadaver study. Clin Anat. 2008;21(7):666–73.
15. Ozgur BM, Aryan HE, Pimenta L, Taylor WR. Extreme lateral interbody fusion (XLIF): a novel surgical technique for anterior lumbar interbody fusion. Spine J. 2006;6(4):435–43.
16. Sclafani JA, Kim CW. Complications associated with the initial learning curve of minimally invasive spine surgery: a systematic review. Clin Orthop Relat Res. 2014;472(6):1711–7.
17. Rodgers WB, Gerber EJ, Patterson J. Intraoperative and early postoperative complications in extreme lateral interbody fusion: an analysis of 600 cases. Spine. 2011;36(1):26–32.

18. Yen CP, Uribe JS, et al. Spine (Phila Pa 1976). 2016;41(Suppl 8):S152–8.
19. Mogannam A, Bianchi C, Chiriano J, Patel S, Teruya TH, Lum SS, et al. Effects of prior abdominal surgery, obesity, and lumbar spine level on anterior retroperitoneal exposure of the lumbar spine. Arch Surg. 2012;147(12):1130–4.
20. Molinares DM, Davis TT, Fung DA. Retroperitoneal oblique corridor to the L2-S1 intervertebral discs: an MRI study. J Neurosurg Spine. 2016;24(2):248–55.
21. Orita S, Inage K, Sainoh T, Fujimoto K, Sato J, Shiga Y, et al. Lower lumbar segmental arteries can intersect over the intervertebral disc in the oblique lateral interbody fusion approach with a risk for arterial injury: radiological analysis of lumbar segmental arteries by using magnetic resonance imaging. Spine. 2017;42(3):135–42.
22. Davis TT, Hynes RA, Fung DA, Spann SW, MacMillan M, Kwon B, et al. Retroperitoneal oblique corridor to the L2-S1 intervertebral discs in the lateral position: an anatomic study. J Neurosurg Spine. 2014;21(5):785–93.
23. Uribe JS, Arredondo N, Dakwar E, Vale FL. Defining the safe working zones using the minimally invasive lateral retroperitoneal transpsoas approach: an anatomical study. J Neurosurg Spine. 2010;13(2):260–6.
24. Chung NS, Jeon CH, Lee HD, Kweon HJ. Preoperative evaluation of left common iliac vein in oblique lateral interbody fusion at L5-S1. Eur Spine J. 2017;26:2797.
25. Beckman JM, Vincent B, Park MS, Billys JB, Isaacs RE, Pimenta L, et al. Contralateral psoas hematoma after minimally invasive, lateral retroperitoneal transpsoas lumbar interbody fusion: a multicenter review of 3950 lumbar levels. J Neurosurg Spine. 2017;26(1):50–4.
26. Uribe JS, Harris JE, Beckman JM, Turner AW, Mundis GM, Akbarnia BA. Finite element analysis of lordosis restoration with anterior longitudinal ligament release and lateral hyperlordotic cage placement. Eur Spine J. 2015;24(Suppl 3):420–6.
27. Chang J, Kim JS, Jo H. Ventral dural injury after oblique lumbar interbody fusion. World Neurosurg. 2017;98:881.e1–4.

Chapter 9
Percutaneous Pedicle Screw/Rod Fixation

Daniel Serban, Niki Calina, Anthony DiGiorgio, Lindsay Lasseigne, and Gabriel Tender

Introduction

Percutaneous instrumented posterior fixation with pedicle screws and rods is one of the most commonly used minimally invasive techniques. The insertion of the percutaneous pedicle screws is identical among the various platforms, whereas insertion of the rod can be done in three different ways, depending on the system utilized.

Indications

The common indications for the percutaneous pedicle screw/rod fixation are outlined below:

- The contralateral side after a minimally invasive transforaminal lumbar interbody fusion (MI TLIF)
- Unilateral or bilateral fixation after lateral (XLIF) or anterior (ALIF, Axialif) lumbar arthrodesis

---

Electronic Supplementary Material The online version of this chapter https://doi.org/10.1007/978-3-319-71943-6_9. contains supplementary material, which is available to authorized users.

D. Serban • N. Calina
Department of Neurosurgery, "Bagdasar-Arseni" Hospital, Bucharest, Romania

A. DiGiorgio • L. Lasseigne
Department of Neurosurgery, Louisiana State University Health Sciences Center, New Orleans, LA, USA
e-mail: Adigi2@lsuhsc.edu; llasse@lsuhsc.edu

G. Tender (✉)
Louisiana State University, New Orleans, LA, USA

G. Tender (ed.), *Minimally Invasive Spine Surgery Techniques*,
https://doi.org/10.1007/978-3-319-71943-6_9

- Trauma: Bilateral fixation after corpectomy and cage insertion (thoracic or lumbar)
- Trauma: Temporary fixation in comminuted vertebral body fractures (thoracic or lumbar) that are likely to heal in 3–6 months with immobilization, but are too unstable to be treated by bracing alone.

Contraindications

Contraindications are relative and include:

- Inability to adequately visualize bony anatomy with the C-arm
- Severe osteoporosis
- Extensive disruption of bony anatomy, such as in: severe deformity, high-grade spondylolisthesis, or prior postero-lateral fusion
- Tumor or infection at the instrumented level

Surgical Technique

Pedicle Screw Insertion

The patient is placed in prone position with the arms tucked to the sides and with adequate padding for all pressure points.

The accurate placement of the pedicle screws is dependent of the quality of the radiologic images. Therefore, obtaining true AP and lateral images prior to skin incision is of utmost importance.

The AP image should be obtained first. The C-arm is locked at 90°, perfectly centered on the vertebral body of interest. This is particularly important if the patient has significant deformity, in which case the C-arm should be readjusted for each vertebral body. The spinous process of the vertebral body of interest should be centered between the two pedicle rings; otherwise, the table (NOT the C-arm) should be tilted left or right until the desired position is achieved. Then, the table is placed either in Trendelenburg or reverse Trendelenburg until the superior endplate of the vertebral body of interest becomes a single line.

The lateral image is obtained next. If the AP image was perfect, now the posterior margin of the targeted vertebral body should appear as a single line. The perfect lateral image is obtained by "wagging" the C-arm until the two pedicles of the vertebral body of interest overlap. At this point, the superior and inferior endplates should also appear as a single line.

After this, the bony landmarks can be marked on patient's skin under AP fluoroscopy: the midline, the left and right pedicle lines, and the interpedicular line for the

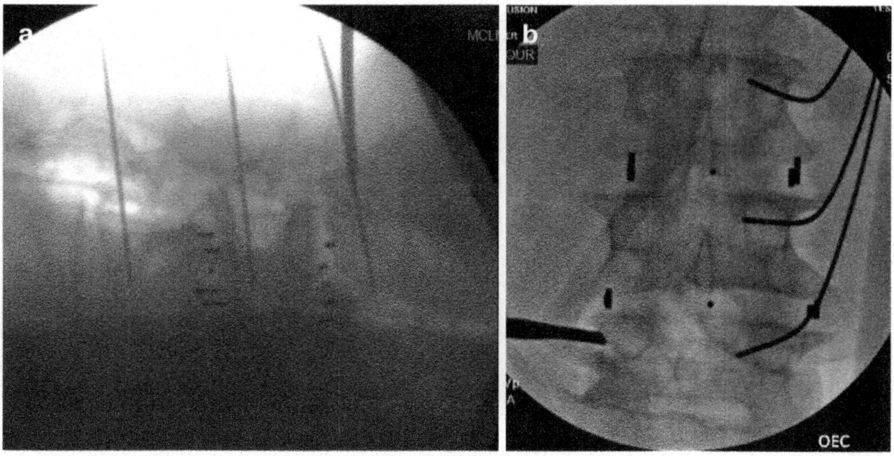

Fig. 9.1 AP and lateral intraoperative images illustrating the ideal initial position of the Jamshidi needle. (**a**) The lateral image shows the tip of the needle just above the transverse process. (**b**) The AP image shows the tip of the needle just outside the pedicle ring

vertebral body of interest. The skin incision should be about 2 cm in length, vertical and centered on the interpedicular line, about 4–6 cm off the midline. This point is typically at or just lateral to the tip of the transverse process on the AP image. In large patients, the skin incision has to be made further lateral, in order to maintain the same lateral-to-medial angle of insertion.

The lumbar fascia is then incised with the knife medial to the skin incision. It is important to remember that the fascia is the layer that limits the exploration of the deep bony landmarks. Continuing in the same lateral to medial direction, the index finger can be inserted to find the junction between the transverse process and the lateral facet. Typically, the lateral facet is first encountered (since it is the most superficial), and then the finger is allowed to slide lateral to it and land on the posterior aspect of the transverse process. If the incision is too small to accommodate a finger, the same landmarks can be identified with the tip of a Jamshidi needle, with the aid of frequent fluoroscopic images. The ideal docking point is at the junction of the transverse process with the lateral facet, as medial as allowed by the lateral facet. On the AP image, this point will appear just outside the pedicle ring (Fig. 9.1); if it appears inside the pedicle ring, it is likely that the tip of the needle is actually riding high on the lateral facet, not on the transverse process (Fig. 9.2). On the lateral image, the tip of the needle should be just above the ring of the transverse process, not high on the lateral facet, and the trajectory should pass through the pedicle, parallel to the endplates. If fine adjustments are necessary, the tip of the Jamshidi needle can be moved with both hands (for maximal control) in millimeter increments, on the base of the transverse process, until the desired position is achieved.

Once the correct docking point is obtained, the needle is gently tapped through the pedicle. For the lower lumbar pedicles, the direction is typically lateral to medial

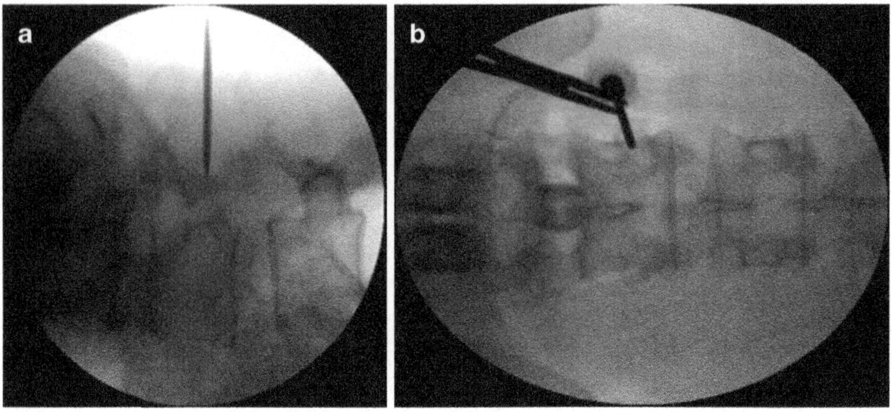

Fig. 9.2 AP and lateral intraoperative images illustrating the incorrect initial position of the Jamshidi needle. (**a**) The lateral image shows the tip of the needle high on the lamina. (**b**) The AP image shows the tip of the needle inside the pedicle ring

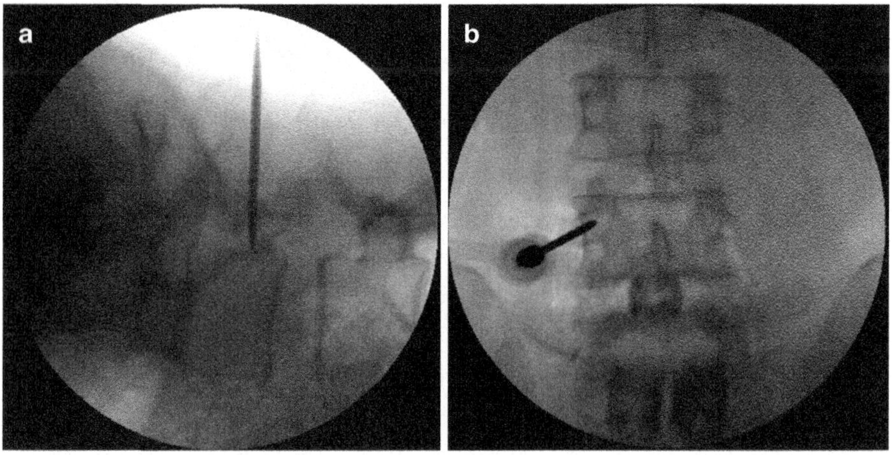

Fig. 9.3 AP and lateral intraoperative images illustrating the most important position of the Jamshidi needle. (**a**) The lateral image shows the tip of the needle at the base of the pedicle. (**b**) The AP image shows the tip of the needle well inside the pedicle ring, but not too close to the medial border

and cranial to caudal, but the angles vary with each level (see below). As the needle is advanced through the pedicle, there should be no increased resistance (that would signify cortical bone and therefore imminent pedicle wall breach). The most important images are obtained when the tip of the needle reaches the base of the pedicle on the lateral image; at this time, the tip of the needle should be still within the pedicle ring on the AP image (Fig. 9.3).

At this time, neuromonitoring is usually employed. The shaft of the needle is stimulated, and a response of 10 mA or above signifies that the medial or inferior pedicle walls have not been breached.

A particular situation is encountered if the tip of the needle is very close to the medial border of the pedicle ring on the AP image, and neuromonitoring yields low responses (e.g., 4–7 mA). In this situation, it is likely that the needle has violated the lateral recess, which sometimes loops under the line of the pedicle ring. Therefore, it is recommended that the tip of the needle should be well within the pedicle ring on the AP images, when it reaches the base of the pedicle on the lateral images.

Another important technical tool is changing the direction of the Jamshidi needle while in the pedicle. Indeed, if the original trajectory is angled too much lateral to medial, and the tip of the needle gets too close to the medial border of the pedicle on the AP image, the angulation of the needle can be changed to a more straight trajectory, without withdrawing the needle from the pedicle. The angulation can also be changed in a cranio-caudal direction, in order to keep the needle parallel to the endplates. Beveled needles are particularly useful in this situation, since they naturally change direction depending on the bevel orientation.

Once the needle trajectory is deemed safe, the tip of the needle is advanced into the vertebral body for a couple of centimeters, and then the center part of the needle is removed and a K-wire is inserted for about another centimeter past the tip of the Jamshidi needle, in order to stabilize it to the cancellous bone and make it less likely to inadvertently come out during the placement of the tap and screw. Then, the Jamshidi needle is removed, while the K-wire is kept in place with the other hand.

After this, most systems have a series of tubular dilators that slide over the K-wire; the outer dilator and the K-wire are kept in place, whereas the inner dilators are removed to make room for the tap and screw. The tap is then advanced over the K-wire into the pedicle of the vertebral body; it is sufficient (and recommended) to tap only past the base of the pedicle and not all the way into the vertebral body. For biomechanical reasons, we recommend undertapping by 2 mm (i.e., use a 4.5 mm tap for a 6.5 mm screw), in order to maintain the good purchase of the screw into the bone. It is important to maintain the direction of the K-wire with the tap; if the tap is not aligned with the K-wire, the part of the K-wire in the vertebral body starts to bend at the tip of the tap, and when a critical angle is reached, the tap cannot advance any more, and any further turns of the tap do nothing but strip (and destroy) the pedicle.

The tap is then removed and the screw (typically 6.5 × 45 mm for the average person) is inserted over the K-wire. Once the tip of the screw passes the base of the pedicle, the K-wire can be removed, and the screw further inserted through the previously created trajectory. The screw insertion must stop just before the head of the screw abuts the lateral facet; otherwise, the screw head loses its' poliaxial capabilities and makes subsequent rod insertion more difficult. All the screws have extender blades attached to their heads, in order to facilitate rod placement.

Insertion of Subsequent Pedicle Screws

Of course, at least 2 pedicle screws per side have to be inserted. The described technique is changed in the fact that most surgeons choose to insert all the K-wires in their respective pedicles before performing the tapping and screw insertion. A useful trick, particularly at L5–S1, is to perform the dissection with the index finger by moving it from the entry point of L5 to the entry point of S1; this also creates a working plane over which the rod can be easily inserted. In patients requiring long constructs (e.g., for trauma fixation, or in deformity correction), it is extremely important to be consistent with the docking point for each level, since the junctions between the transverse process and the lateral facet are lined up in a cranio-caudal fashion. If one of the insertion points was too medial or too lateral, it will not align with the rest. In this case, if trying to reduce the rod to that screw head fails, the only option is to remove that pedicle screw and skip that level, since most pedicles are not large enough to accommodate two separate 6.5 mm screw channels (exception: the S1 pedicle, which is large enough to accommodate more than one trajectory).

In long constructs, most systems allow for determining the rod sizing and contouring prior to its' insertion, by reproducing at skin level the height of the screw heads.

Individual Lumbar Levels

S1. The S1 pedicle is the largest. The transverse process equivalent in the sacrum is the ala, so the docking point for this level is found at the junction between the sacral facet and the ala. On the routine AP image, the tip of the needle will appear cranial and lateral to the pedicle ring, and just outside of it. On the lateral image, it will appear somewhat caudal. Since the pedicle is so large, there are a couple of options in choosing the entry point. One option involves starting the pedicle cannulation close to its cranial aspect and keeping the trajectory parallel to the endplate; this is the usual placement of screws ipsilateral to an MI TLIF construct, where the entry point is already exposed. The other option involves starting the cannulation more caudally and aim towards the sacral promontorium; this option is used when the distance between the L5 and S1 screw heads needs to be wider (e.g., for performing an MI TLIF using the pedicle-based retractor technique). It also allows for insertion of longer screws with better bone purchase, since the sacral lip has extremely hard bone.

The S1 pedicle is typically cannulated at 30° in the lateral-medial direction and about 30–60° in the cranial to caudal direction (this angle varies with the sacral tilt).

L5. The L5 pedicle is probably the hardest to cannulate, due to its small size and often sclerotic bone, as well as the fact that the pedicle image is partially masked by the iliac crest on the lateral X-ray. The docking point is usually close to the S1 one, and we prefer to place the L5 pedicle screw as cranial in the pedicle as possible, not only to avoid damage to the L5 spinal nerve wrapping around the infero-medial aspect of the pedicle, but also to offer more space between the L5 and S1 pedicle screw heads (e.g., for an MI TLIF using the pedicle-based retractor technique).

The L5 pedicle is typically cannulated at 25–30° in the lateral-medial direction and 10–20° in the cranial to caudal direction.

L4. The L4 pedicle is usually larger than L5 and easy to identify on the lateral image. The L4 pedicle is typically cannulated at about 15–20° in the lateral-medial direction and close to 0° ("straight down") in the cranial to caudal direction.

L3–L1. These pedicles are oriented in an almost sagittal position (5–15° lateral to medial), with increasing caudal to cranial angles, due to the normal lordotic curve of the lumbar spine. At these levels, the skin incision has to be closer to the midline, at about 3–4 cm.

Rod Insertion

Rod insertion can be done in three different ways, depending on the system.

The first way involves inserting the rod through a separate stab wound (e.g., Sextant/Longitude of Medtronic). One of the advantages of these systems is that it preserves the fascia and soft tissues between the towers. Another advantage (Sextant) is that it provides the most precise spondylolisthesis reduction. Finally, the Longitude system may provide easier navigation of the rod through the multiple towers. The main disadvantage of Sextant is that 2-level fixation is difficult (and 3-level is almost impossible). Another disadvantage is the additional skin incisions made for rod insertion.

The second way involves inserting the rod through either the cranial or the caudal tower (e.g., Revolve of Globus, ES2 of Stryker, Viper of Depuy-Acromed, Serengeti of K2M). The advantage is that it does not need an additional skin incision. The disadvantage is that it is somewhat more difficult to pass through all the towers, particularly in multilevel cases.

The third way involves dropping the rod through the towers (e.g., Spherx DBR of Nuvasive). This can only be done for a maximum of 2-level fusions. The disadvantage is that the tissues between the towers have to be disrupted; however, these tissues are already violated during screw placement. The advantage is that the rod has no overhang, and therefore the adjacent joints (particularly the cranial one) are somewhat protected from further degeneration (at least theoretically).

Regardless of the insertion method, the rod is then locked to the screw heads with appropriate caps. Most current systems have built-in reduction capabilities, which preclude the need for persuaders and can be used to reduce deformity curves. Once the rod is locked in place, the towers are removed from the screw heads and the wounds are closed in layers.

Tricks and Pitfalls

The AP Insertion Technique

This technique is a shortcut that should not be used by beginners. In patients requiring long constructs, in order to save time and not have to go back and forth between AP and lateral images, the pedicle screws can be inserted under AP imaging only [1] (Video 9.1). The docking point for each level is selected as previously described, based on palpation and AP imaging. Once the tip of the needle is engaged in the bone, a mark is placed on the needle at 2 cm from the skin level. This corresponds to the normal length of the pedicle. The Jamshidi needle is then advanced into the pedicle until the mark reaches the skin level, i.e., the tip of the needle is at the base of the pedicle. At this time, the AP image should show the tip of the needle still within the ring of the pedicle. The needle is then advanced further into the vertebral body and then used to place the K-wire in the respective pedicle. This technique implies that the surgeon knows the angles of insertion for each pedicle, as well as the direction of the endplates.

The Bicortical Technique

This technique is occasionally necessary for patients with osteoporosis or when reduction of a spondylolisthesis on pedicle screws is planned, when increased screw pullout strength is needed. The pedicle is cannulated as previously described, and a K-wire is inserted. The tap is then driven all the way to the anterior cortex of the vertebral body; if the tap is aggressive enough (i.e., if the tip is sharp enough, depending on the system), the tap can be advanced through the anterior cortex. Otherwise, the tap is removed, and the Jamshidi needle is reinserted over the K-wire and then tapped gently through the anterior cortex. Extreme care must be exercised after this maneuver, since the tip of the K-wire must not be pushed past the anterior cortex (and potentially injure the great vessels in the abdomen), but also not pulled out of the pedicle and lose the cannulated path. "Safe" wires (with a "Y" split as they are inserted through the Jamshidi needle) can be used in these cases to prevent injury of the abdominal vessels. The pedicle screw (with the attached tower) is then advanced over the K-wire all the way to and then through the anterior vertebral body cortex. Obviously, the pedicle screw length has to be determined prior to its insertion and has to span the distance between the entry point and the anterior cortex (usually 55–65 mm).

Changing of Trajectory with the Tap Over the K-Wire

This technical trick can be used when the Jamshidi needle and K-wire were inserted very close to the medial or inferior border of the pedicle and there is concern that placing the wider tap and screw over that trajectory might lead to a breach of the respective wall. In this situation, the tap is intentionally directed at an angle with the K-wire, in the more desirable trajectory. Once the tap reaches the base of the pedicle, the K-wire is pulled out and the tap is further advanced into the vertebral body. Finally, the K-wire is reinserted through the tap into the new, more desirable position.

Monitoring the Needle During Insertion

Some companies offer continuous neuromonitoring feedback during needle insertion. One of them is Nuvasive: a clip is attached to the shaft of the needle, and an isolating sleeve allows only the tip to be monitored by electromyography. The numbers displayed must stay above 10 mA in order for the insertion to be considered safe. Another company is Pediguard: there is auditory feedback as the needle is advanced through the pedicle, and approaching the cortical bone of the pedicle yields high-pitched sounds before the pedicle wall is breached.

Complications

Misplacement

This is the most obvious and common complication. Usually, the tap violates the medial cortex at the base of the pedicle, contacting the exiting spinal nerve in the lateral recess. This is signaled by the low numbers obtained on neurostimulation, usually less than 5 mA. In this case, depending on the size of the pedicle, the surgeon can try to place a new entry point and create a new trajectory in the pedicle; however, since the medial cortex has been breached, neurostimulation will always yield low numbers, even if the tap/pedicle screw are now well within the pedicle. Therefore, the surgeon has only the AP and lateral fluoroscopy to rely on during the new trajectory creation.

Occasionally, the pedicle screw is inserted too lateral, outside the vertebral body. This is usually detected postoperatively, if a CT scan is performed. If the patient is asymptomatic (i.e., no radiculopathy) and the screw does not violate the vascular structures, no revision is necessary, as long as the stability of the construct is good. Patients with concordant radiculopathy are, of course, re-explored, and the misplaced screw is removed. If the pedicle is small and does not allow insertion of a screw with a new trajectory, we occasionally use the "cortical screw" trajectory. The entry point is more medial, on the pars interarticularis, and the trajectory is "up and out", similar to the lateral mass screws in the cervical spine. The screws are typically shorter and exit the vertebral body laterally, just cranial to the pedicle. This variation works in one or two level fusions, since the rod can be adequately bent, but does not work in longer constructs, as the screw head is medial and will not line up with the rest of the screw heads above and below; in these cases, we recommend simply leaving that screw out.

Loosening or Breakage

These complications usually follow pseudarthrosis. The revision has to take into account not only the screw replacement or removal, but also adding a fusion surface. Depending on the initial type of fusion performed, the revision may involve a different type of interbody grafting and/or a postero-lateral, intertransverse, fusion. If the pedicle has been destroyed by the loose screw, and if the "cortical screw" trajectory is not feasible, additional cranial and/or caudal levels may have to be involved in the fusion.

Some of these cases require conversion to an open exposure (e.g., converting to the cortical trajectory or extending the fusion over multiple levels). In these cases, if the screws have to be removed, it may be necessary to re-open the initial incisions, in order to be able to gain the same angle for the screwdriver. For this particular reason, we prefer to "medialize" the screw heads before locking the rods in place, so that they can be easier to access in case an open approach may become necessary in the future.

Cranial Facet Joint Violation

The cranial pedicle screws in any construct are, by default, situated next to a joint that will continue to be mobile. The percutaneous pedicle screws have a starting point at the angle between the lateral facet and transverse process, and therefore are farther from the joint than the open pedicle screws, which are typically started slightly more medial, on the lateral facet. Moreover, in open cases, the capsule of the cranial facet joint is sometimes inadvertently violated during the exposure, which increases the risk of adjacent level disease.

Literature Review

The safety of lumbar percutaneous pedicle screw insertion has been shown to be similar to that of open pedicle screws [2, 3]. Most studies report a low incidence of percutaneous pedicle screw misplacement (greater than 95% accuracy [2]); moreover, these misplaced screws rarely result in symptoms and require revision [2, 4–7]. Out of 601 percutaneously placed screws performed for MI TLIF, Smith et al. found only two symptomatic pedicle breaches [6]. Hansen-Algenstaedt et al. found that the highest pedicle breach rates were at T1, T4 & S1 [7].

The cranial facet joint violation can occur with percutaneous pedicle screws, just as it does with open cases. However, the literature is ambivalent, some studies favoring the percutaneous pedicle screws [8, 9], while others suggest the opposite [10, 11]. Wang et al. found no difference in the rates in a meta-analysis incorporating 1755 cranial pedicle screws [8]. Yson et al. favored the percutanoues technique in 370 screws, with a significantly higher chance of facet violation as one progresses from L1–L5. Babu et al. and Park et al. favored open screws in two smaller studies (279 screws and 184 screws, respectively) [10, 11].

Conclusions

Percutaneous pedicle screw insertion technique is useful for posterior lumbar stabilization with minimal morbidity.

References

1. Ahmad FU, Wang MY. Use of anteroposterior view fluoroscopy for targeting percutaneous pedicle screws in cases of spinal deformity with axial rotation. J Neurosurg Spine. 2014;21:826–32. https://doi.org/10.3171/2014.7.spine13846.
2. Ikeuchi H, Ikuta K. Accuracy of pedicle screw insertion in the thoracic and lumbar spine: a comparative study between percutaneous screw insertion and conventional open technique. Arch Orthop Trauma Surg. 2016;136:1195–202. https://doi.org/10.1007/s00402-016-2502-0.
3. Oh HS, Kim JS, Lee SH, Liu WC, Hong SW. Comparison between the accuracy of percutaneous and open pedicle screw fixations in lumbosacral fusion. Spine J. 2013;13:1751–7. https://doi.org/10.1016/j.spinee.2013.03.042.
4. Chiu CK, Kwan MK, Chan CY, Schaefer C, Hansen-Algenstaedt N. The accuracy and safety of fluoroscopically guided percutaneous pedicle screws in the lumbosacral junction and the lumbar spine: a review of 880 screws. Bone Joint J. 2015;97-B:1111–7. https://doi.org/10.1302/0301-620x.97b8.35330.
5. Nimjee SM, et al. Safe and accurate placement of thoracic and thoracolumbar percutaneous pedicle screws without image-navigation. Asian J Neurosurg. 2015;10:272–5. https://doi.org/10.4103/1793-5482.162700.
6. Smith ZA, Sugimoto K, Lawton CD, Fessler RG. Incidence of lumbar spine pedicle breach after percutaneous screw fixation: a radiographic evaluation of 601 screws in 151 patients. J Spinal Disord Tech. 2014;27:358–63. https://doi.org/10.1097/BSD.0b013e31826226cb.
7. Hansen-Algenstaedt N, et al. Accuracy and safety of fluoroscopic guided percutaneous pedicle screws in thoracic and lumbosacral spine: a review of 2000 screws. Spine. 2015;40:E954–63. https://doi.org/10.1097/brs.0000000000000958.
8. Wang L, Wang Y, Yu B, Li Z, Li Y. Comparison of cranial facet joint violation rate between percutaneous and open pedicle screw placement: a systematic review and meta-analysis. Medicine. 2015;94:e504. https://doi.org/10.1097/md.0000000000000504.
9. Yson SC, et al. Comparison of cranial facet joint violation rates between open and percutaneous pedicle screw placement using intraoperative 3-D CT (O-arm) computer navigation. Spine. 2013;38:E251–8. https://doi.org/10.1097/BRS.0b013e31827ecbf1.
10. Babu R, et al. Comparison of superior-level facet joint violations during open and percutaneous pedicle screw placement. Neurosurgery. 2012;71:962–70. https://doi.org/10.1227/NEU.0b013e31826a88c8.
11. Park Y, Ha JW, Lee YT, Sung NY. Cranial facet joint violations by percutaneously placed pedicle screws adjacent to a minimally invasive lumbar spinal fusion. Spine J. 2011;11:295–302. https://doi.org/10.1016/j.spinee.2011.02.007.

Chapter 10
The Presacral Approach (AxiaLIF)

John Gachiani, Silvia Gesheva, Mihaela Florea, and Gabriel Tender

Introduction

The presacral approach (AxiaLIF) offers a minimally invasive fusion option for the L5–S1 (or the L4–L5 and L5–S1) discs, taking advantage of the presacral space and transsacral trajectory. Supplemental posterior stabilization with either percutaneous facet or pedicle screws is indicated, in order to limit rotation. While we believe this is a great procedure for selected patients, the implants have become difficult to obtain, due in part to multiple changes in company ownership.

Surgical Anatomy

The presacral approach takes advantage of a relatively "bare" area, a virtual space between the parietal fascia, covering the anterior surface of the sacrum and the presacral vessels and sympathetic trunk, and the visceral fascia,

---

Electronic Supplementary Material The online version of this chapter https://doi.org/10.1007/978-3-319-71943-6_10. contains supplementary material, which is available to authorized users.

J. Gachiani
Mercy Neurosurgery, Des Moines, IA, USA

S. Gesheva
Department of Neurosurgery, Louisiana State University Health Sciences Center, New Orleans, LA, USA
e-mail: sgeshe@lsuhsc.edu

M. Florea
Department of Neurosurgery, "Bagdasar-Arseni" Hospital, Bucharest, Romania

G. Tender (✉)
Louisiana State University, New Orleans, LA, USA

G. Tender (ed.), *Minimally Invasive Spine Surgery Techniques*,
https://doi.org/10.1007/978-3-319-71943-6_10

covering the rectum. This virtual space contains loose areolar tissue and fat. The vessels on the anterior surface of the sacrum include the middle sacral artery as well as a venous plexus, anastomozing in a stair-like fashion. The pelvic splanchnic nerves originate from the anterior branches of the S2–S4 nerves and pierce the parietal presacral fascia at the lateral sacral foramens to join the hypogastric nerve on the pelvic wall and form the inferior hypogastric plexus, closely adherent to the rectum.

Biomechanics

The biomechanical analysis of the AxiaLIF construct has been previously described. The superior end of the AxiaLIF rod has been designed to have a conic shape in order to prevent subsidence upon axial loading. However, the vertical position of the axial rod, combined with its round shape, lead to relatively low resistance of the construct to axial rotation. Therefore, it is mandatory that the axial rod fixation is supplemented with posterior fixation (either facet or pedicle screws) in order to limit rotation.

Indications

The patients selected to undergo the AxiaLIF lumbosacral fusion are similar to the candidates for any other type of fusion (PLIF, TLIF, or ALIF). We use the Fritzell criteria for patient selection: at least 2 years history of intractable low back pain, failed conservative management (including at least 3 months of physical therapy), and pathology limited to the L5–S1 segment. The type of L5–S1 pathology is typically the degenerative disc disease, including collapsed disc space, Modic changes in the adjacent endplates, anterior and posterior osteophytes, and facet hypertrophy. Other common indications for the AxiaLIF technique include: L5–S1 disease after previous laminectomy and/or discectomy, L5–S1 grade I or II spondylolisthesis, and L5–S1 fusion for anterior support in long fusions to the sacrum for scoliosis.

Contraindications

The three common contraindications are: abnormal sacral anatomy (flat or hooked sacrum), insufficient presacral fat pad, and large, anomalous presacral vessels. These anatomic variations have a low incidence and can be easily identified on a preoperative MRI that includes the tip of the sacrum.

Preoperative Planning

The most important radiologic investigation is the MRI of the lower lumbar spine to include the tip of the sacrum. The MRI shows the shape of the sacrum and allows for trajectory planning, from the paracoccygeal notch to the mid-body of L5; if the patient has a hooked or flat sacrum, this trajectory is usually not feasible. The sagittal T2-weighted MRI also shows the presacral fat pad and may point to scarring due to prior operations in the area (e.g., rectal resection or radiation). Finally, the MRI may show large anomalous presacral vessels as flow voids on the sagittal T2-weighted images.

Flexion-extension radiographs may help in determining the mobility of an L5–S1 spondylolisthesis, and computed tomography may assist in determining the integrity of the L5 pars interarticularis (particularly in patients with spondylolisthesis).

Other preoperative measures include a standard bowel prep the day before the surgery (similar to that for a colonoscopy) and gram negative and anaerobic antibiotic coverage 1 h prior to the skin incision. Informed consents should include an alternative fusion method, in case of intraoperative difficulties.

Surgical Technique

Positioning

The patient is placed in prone position on a Wilson frame or similar, with enough room under patient's pelvis to accommodate the AP C-arm (Video 10.1). The Wilson frame is used so that enough working room is ensured to "drop the hand" during the blunt presacral dissection. The buttocks are taped in adducted position, a towel soaked in betadine is inserted in the anus, and an adhesive drape is placed over the anus to isolate it from the operative field.

Two C-arms are placed in lateral and AP positions, respectively, in a set up similar to that of a vertebroplasty. The lateral C-arm is placed under the table and then rotated cranially to allow for positioning of the AP C-arm from the same side of the patient and at about 45° angle with the patient. The 2 C-arms are centered on the L5–S1 disc space.

Access to the Presacral Space

The coccygeal tip is felt through the skin, as well as the paracoccygeal notch (the sacro-spinous ligament). The skin incision is about 2 cm long, 1 cm off the midline and just below the notch. The sharp dissection can be continued to the first layer of paracoccygeal fascia, but no deeper than the bony layer. Further dissection through the layers of fascia has to be done bluntly, preferably with the finger, or alternatively with a curved Kelly clamp. The complete fascial penetration is typically perceived as a sudden loss of resistance (a "pop"), and the tactile feel is that of the shiny smooth anterior surface of the sacrum. Dissection in this plane very easy and feels like loose areolar tissue (like "cotton candy").

Once the anterior surface of the sacrum is felt with the tip of the index finger, further dissection is done with the blunt obturator, with slow advancement under bilateral fluoroscopic guidance. The tip of the obturator should be maintained against the bone surface, but without pushing too hard, in order to protect the venous plexus underneath the parietal fascia. If the tip of the obturator feels blocked, it can be either the "bump" of a vestigial disc, or it may be too lateral, in the sacral foramen (easily identified on the AP fluoroscopy). The dissection should be carried out past the docking point, in order to prevent bowel injuries at the time of the outer cannula insertion. The ideal docking point is slightly off to the side of the incision and perpendicular to the L5–S1 disc on both the AP and lateral fluoroscopic images. The imaginary line along the obturator should cross the L5–S1 disc slightly posterior to its center on the lateral image.

Final AP and lateral images should be obtained just before inserting the guide pin, since the obturator can move upon removal of its center part (in which case the obturator should be reassembled before moving it). The bevel of the guide pin can be used to adjust the trajectory in the sacrum. Further adjusting can be performed when drilling through the sacrum.

Discectomy

The radial cutters (looped or flat) are used to detach the nucleus from the endplates. This is easier to accomplish if the direction of the cutters is perfectly perpendicular to the L5–S1 disc on the AP image. The largest feasible discectomy should be pursued. Obviously, the cutters should not go posteriorly past the annulus fibrosus, in order to avoid a dural laceration. Ideally, the endplates of both L5 and S1 should be circumferentially denuded (which gives a typical feel and rasping noise). However, special attention should be paid not to "dig holes" in the endplates with the aggressive cutter.

Grafting

Typically, about 10 cm^3 of graft material can be then directionally inserted into the disc space. When enough material is inserted, it becomes difficult to advance the tip of the inserter into the disc space.

Fixation and Distraction

Before advancing in the L5 vertebral body with the drill, lordosis can be restored by raising the hand holding the drill. A decision has to be made whether distraction is necessary. We prefer to have rods with either zero or minimal (1–2 mm) distraction, in order not to loosen the graft and allow for Wolff's law to promote the fusion.

Closure

We close the wound in anatomical layers with 2-0 Vycril on a UR5 needle for the paracoccygeal fascia, then interrupted 3-0 Vycril for the hypodermis and 4-0 Monocryl subcuticular and Dermabond or other liquid bonding agents for the skin.

Tricks and Pitfalls

Spondylolisthesis

We have previously described the technique for spondylolisthesis treatment using the AxiaLIF [1]. The pedicle screws at L5 and S1 are inserted in a bicortical fashion, particularly at L5, since we rely on their pullout strength to reduce the spondylolisthesis. The pedicle screw system must be designed to have the capability of spondylolisthesis reduction (e.g., the CD Horizon Sextant system, Medtronic, Sofamor Danek, Memphis, TN). Once the screws are in place, the rods are locked on the screw heads of S1 bilaterally, at an angle commensurate with the need for reduction. There is a slight lag before the reduction starts, so, if a 1 cm reduction is needed, the rod is left about 1.4 cm proud on the L5 head. Most systems allow for up to 2 cm reduction, which normally corresponds to grades 1 or 2 spondylolisthesis. Then, the caps are placed through the L5 towers and the rods are gradually and simultaneously brought onto the L5 screw heads, thus reducing the spondylolisthesis. There is a potential risk of stripping the pedicles (e.g., in patients with osteoporosis and poor bone purchase by the pedicle screw), but we have not encountered this complication yet. As the spondylolisthesis is reduced, the L5–S1 interspace is typically also distracted ("opened up"). After spondylolisthesis reduction, the L5 caps are not locked onto the rods yet, still allowing for a translational movement.

The presacral approach is then performed. Since the spondylolisthesis was reduced, the trajectory of the axial rod should now be feasible. Therefore, a 2 cm paracoccygeal skin incision was made and the presacral approach was performed to place the anterior axial rod. The trajectory can be adjusted by turning the bevel of the guide pin in the desired direction as it is advanced through the sacrum. After the discectomy, a large amount of graft is inserted in the interspace, and then the axial rod is advanced through S1 into L5. Further distraction of the L5–S1 interspace can be performed, if needed, but that will also result in some loosening of the bone graft; therefore, we prefer to add no or minimal extra-distraction with the axial rod.

Once the axial rod is in the desired position, the caps are locked on the rods and the towers are removed. The three small wounds are closed in anatomical layers. This technique offers a biomechanical advantage, when compared to the TLIF or ALIF interbody devices, in that the axial rod directly opposes the sheer forces of spondylolisthesis and thus potentially prevents construct failure.

Complications

Bowel Injury

This is the most feared complication by the spine surgeons, who are not accustomed to operate around bowels. Nonetheless, the incidence of bowel injuries with AxiaLIF is very low. Treatment of bowel injuries typically involve a temporary colostomy, although superficial injuries may be treated with primary closure and antibiotics.

Pseudarthrosis

Patients with symptomatic failure of fusion are treated by an alternative method, i.e., ALIF or TLIF/PLIF. The axial rod does not have to be removed unless there is a concomitant infection. We prefer using the PLIF technique for revisions, since it allows placement of two cages in the intervertebral space, one on each side of the axial rod.

Sacral Fracture

This is another rare complication that may occur in patients in which the axial rod was placed too ventral, leaving only a thin rim of bone anterior to the axial rod. The treatment typically involves rod removal and fusion by an alternative method.

Literature Review

The results of this technique have been overall positive [2–6], with high fusion rates and low complication rates. Zeilstra et al. found a 73.8% clinical success rate in 164 patients over 10 years of follow up and an 83% satisfaction rate. Whang et al. found a higher arthrodesis rate and similar complication rate when retrospectively comparing Axialif to ALIF. Hofstetter et al showed an 80% fusion rate at L5–S1 (however, none of the L4–5 levels fused) in a retrospective series of 38 patients.

The literature also reflects the spectrum of somewhat unique complications of this procedure and their treatment [7–13]. These include migration of the cage intraperitonealy, rectal perforation & fistulas and non-unions.

Conclusions

AxiaLIF with pedicle or facet screws offers a minimally invasive alternative for the management of lumbosacral disease. In cases of spondylolisthesis, this technique may have a biomechanical advantage when compared to the traditional ones.

References

1. Tender GC, Miller LE, Block JE. Percutaneous pedicle screw reduction and axial presacral lumbar interbody fusion for treatment of lumbosacral spondylolisthesis: a case series. J Med Case Rep. 2011;5:454. https://doi.org/10.1186/1752-1947-5-454.
2. Zeilstra DJ, Staartjes VE, Schroder ML. Minimally invasive transaxial lumbosacral interbody fusion: a ten year single-centre experience. Int Orthop. 2017;41:113–9. https://doi.org/10.1007/s00264-016-3273-5.
3. Schroeder GD, Kepler CK, Vaccaro AR. Axial interbody arthrodesis of the L5-S1 segment: a systematic review of the literature. J Neurosurg Spine. 2015;23:314–9. https://doi.org/10.3171/2015.1.spine14900.
4. Zeilstra DJ, Miller LE, Block JE. Axial lumbar interbody fusion: a 6-year single-center experience. Clin Interv Aging. 2013;8:1063–9. https://doi.org/10.2147/cia.s49802.
5. Whang PG, Sasso RC, Patel VV, Ali RM, Fischgrund JS. Comparison of axial and anterior interbody fusions of the L5-S1 segment: a retrospective cohort analysis. J Spinal Disord Tech. 2013;26:437–43. https://doi.org/10.1097/BSD.0b013e318292aad7.
6. Hofstetter CP, Shin B, Tsiouris AJ, Elowitz E, Hartl R. Radiographic and clinical outcome after 1- and 2-level transsacral axial interbody fusion: clinical article. J Neurosurg Spine. 2013;19:454–63. https://doi.org/10.3171/2013.6.spine12282.
7. Wilson JR, Timothy J, Rao A, Sagar PM. Retrieval of a migrated AxiaLIF lumbosacral screw using fluoroscopic guidance with simultaneous real-time sigmoidoscopy: technical report. Spine. 2013;38:E1285–7. https://doi.org/10.1097/BRS.0b013e31829fef1b.
8. Siegel G, Patel N, Ramakrishnan R. Rectocutaneous fistula and nonunion after TranS1 axial lumbar interbody fusion L5-S1 fixation: case report. J Neurosurg Spine. 2013;19:197–200. https://doi.org/10.3171/2013.5.spine11523.
9. Mazur MD, Duhon BS, Schmidt MH, Dailey AT. Rectal perforation after AxiaLIF instrumentation: case report and review of the literature. Spine J. 2013;13:e29–34. https://doi.org/10.1016/j.spinee.2013.06.053.
10. Louwerens JK, Groot D, van Duijvenbode DC, Spruit M. Alternative surgical strategy for AxiaLIF pseudarthrosis: a series of three case reports. Evid Based Spine Care J. 2013;4:143–8. https://doi.org/10.1055/s-0033-1357357.
11. Tormenti MJ, et al. Perioperative surgical complications of transforaminal lumbar interbody fusion: a single-center experience. J Neurosurg Spine. 2012;16:44–50. https://doi.org/10.3171/2011.9.SPINE11373.
12. Manjila S, Singer J, Knudson K, Tomac AC, Hart DJ. Minimally invasive presacral retrieval of a failed AxiaLIF rod implant: technical note and illustrative cases. Spine J. 2012;12:940–8. https://doi.org/10.1016/j.spinee.2012.10.026.
13. Lindley EM, McCullough MA, Burger EL, Brown CW, Patel VV. Complications of axial lumbar interbody fusion. J Neurosurg Spine. 2011;15:273–9. https://doi.org/10.3171/2011.3.SPINE10373.

Chapter 11
Percutaneous Facet Screws

Malcolm Daniel Eggart, Silvia Gesheva, Clifford Crutcher, and Gabriel Tender

Introduction

This technique is useful mostly at L4–5 and L5–S1 as supplemental fixation after an anterior approach (ALIF or AxiaLIF) and has the advantage of a minimal midline skin incision and soft tissue disruption. While biomechanically not as strong as the pedicle screw/rod constructs, the facet screws are mostly designed to block rotation.

Indications

The percutaneous facet screws are indicated as supplemental fixation after an anterior approach (ALIF or AxiaLIF), or unilaterally on the contralateral side of an MI TLIF.

Electronic Supplementary Material The online version of this chapter https://doi.org/10.1007/978-3-319-71943-6_11. contains supplementary material, which is available to authorized users.

M.D. Eggart
MUSC Health Neurosciences at Tidelands Health, Murrells Inlet, SC, USA

S. Gesheva • C. Crutcher
Department of Neurosurgery, Louisiana State University Health Sciences Center, New Orleans, LA, USA
e-mail: sgeshe@lsuhsc.edu; ccrutc@lsuhsc.edu

G. Tender (✉)
Louisiana State University, New Orleans, LA, USA

G. Tender (ed.), *Minimally Invasive Spine Surgery Techniques*,
https://doi.org/10.1007/978-3-319-71943-6_11

Contraindications

The higher lumbar levels (L3–4 and above) represent a relative contraindication, due to the smaller size and sagittal orientation of the facet joints.

Surgical Technique

The patient is placed in prone position with the arms tucked to the sides and with adequate padding for all pressure points (Video 11.1). On lateral fluoroscopy, a straight instrument is placed on the side of the patient to evaluate the future trajectory of the facet screws and determine the exact location of the skin incision. A small stab wound (about 1 cm in length) is made, usually between the L3 and L4 spinous processes, and then the underlying lumbar fascia is opened with the 10-blade on both sides of the spinous process in a slightly caudal direction from the skin incision. A beveled Jamshidi-type needle is advanced in the pre-planned cranial to caudal direction, and in a slightly medial to lateral angulation, using the AP fluoroscopic images to direct the tip of the needle. When targeting the L5–S1 facet, the L4 lamina is usually first encountered, and the tip of the needle can be safely navigated over this lamina to land on the L5 pars interarticularis. Before engaging the tip of the needle into the bone, the AP image should show the tip of the needle at the medial pedicular line and the lateral image should show the trajectory of the needle passing just below the intervertebral foramen. The tip of the needle is then gently tapped into the bone, and minor trajectory adjustments can be made by turning the bevel of the needle in the desired direction. A typical loss of resistance is encountered as the tip of the needle crosses the joint. At L5–S1, the needle can be advanced over a longer distance into the S1 pedicle (2–3 cm), whereas at L4–5, the tip of the needle comes out of the lateral side of the L5 pedicle after about 1.5–2 cm. A K-wire is then left in place as the needle is removed, and then a high-speed drill is used to enlarge the path created by the Jamshidi-type needle. A tap can be used in patients with hard bone and then a facet screw is inserted to lock the facet joints (typically 5 × 30 mm for L5–S1 and 2 × 25 mm for L4–5). Optionally, a rasp can be advanced over and lateral to the facet joint to decorticate the outer joint and promote fusion.

Complications

The only unique complication to this technique is misplacement of the facet screw. If the entry point is too medial, the screw may violate the central canal and cauda equina elements, whereas if the entry point is too lateral, the screw may not have enough bony purchase to stabilize the joint. Finally, the screw trajectory may cross the intervertebral foramen, but typically this occurs in the caudal part of the foramen, away from the exiting nerve, and therefore nerve injury/radiculopathy is unlikely.

Literature Review

Percutaneous lumbar facet screws are favored in circumferential fusions, versus pedicle screws, because they offer a comparable biomechanical stiffness and much less blood loss and soft tissue damage [1–5].

Similarly, unilateral facet screws seem to provide advantages over percutaneous pedicle screw fixation in minimally invasive TLIF [6–10].

Conclusions

Lumbar facet screws can be inserted with minimal morbidity in patients who require supplemental posterior fixation.

References

1. Agarwala A, Bucklen B, Muzumdar A, Moldavsky M, Khalil S. Do facet screws provide the required stability in lumbar fixation? A biomechanical comparison of the Boucher technique and pedicular fixation in primary and circumferential fusions. Clin Biomech (Bristol, Avon). 2012;27:64–70. https://doi.org/10.1016/j.clinbiomech.2011.07.007.
2. Best NM, Sasso RC. Efficacy of translaminar facet screw fixation in circumferential interbody fusions as compared to pedicle screw fixation. J Spinal Disord Tech. 2006;19:98–103. https://doi.org/10.1097/01.bsd.0000179244.76244.5e.
3. Buttermann GR, Thorson TM, Mullin WJ. Outcomes of posterior facet versus pedicle screw fixation of circumferential fusion: a cohort study. Eur Spine J. 2014;23:347–55. https://doi.org/10.1007/s00586-013-2999-7.
4. Ferrara LA, et al. A biomechanical comparison of facet screw fixation and pedicle screw fixation: effects of short-term and long-term repetitive cycling. Spine. 2003;28:1226–34. https://doi.org/10.1097/01.brs.0000065485.46539.17.
5. Zhan Y, Tian D. Do translaminar facet screws have the same stability as pedicle screws in two-level anterior lumbar interbody fusion? A biomechanical study. Turk Neurosurg. 2012;22:630–3. https://doi.org/10.5137/1019-5149.jtn.5825-12.0.
6. Awad BI, et al. Bilateral pedicle screw fixation versus unilateral pedicle and contralateral facet screws for minimally invasive transforaminal lumbar interbody fusion: clinical outcomes and cost analysis. Global Spine J. 2013;3:225–30. https://doi.org/10.1055/s-0033-1349399.
7. Cao Y, et al. The combined use of unilateral pedicle screw and contralateral facet joint screw fixation in transforaminal lumbar interbody fusion. Eur Spine J. 2015;24:2607–13. https://doi.org/10.1007/s00586-015-4120-x.
8. Hsiang J, Yu K, He Y. Minimally invasive one-level lumbar decompression and fusion surgery with posterior instrumentation using a combination of pedicle screw fixation and transpedicular facet screw construct. Surg Neurol Int. 2013;4:125. https://doi.org/10.4103/2152-7806.119007.
9. Jang JS, Lee SH. Minimally invasive transforaminal lumbar interbody fusion with ipsilateral pedicle screw and contralateral facet screw fixation. J Neurosurg Spine. 2005;3:218–23. https://doi.org/10.3171/spi.2005.3.3.0218.
10. Luo B, et al. Biomechanical study of unilateral pedicle screw combined with contralateral translaminar facet screw in transforaminal lumbar interbody fusion. Clin Biomech (Bristol, Avon). 2015;30:657–61. https://doi.org/10.1016/j.clinbiomech.2015.05.009.

Chapter 12
Sacro-Iliac Joint Fusion

Gabriel Tender, Alexis Waguespack, Clifford Crutcher, Anthony Digiorgio, and Remi Nader

Introduction

The minimally invasive sacro-iliac joint fusion is a relatively new technique that has been shown to achieve good results. The SI joint is a recently recognized potential pain generator and the diagnosis requires a specific algorithm. The surgeon should always think of this potential source of pain in patients with back pain radiating to one of the legs and no concordant spinal pathology. We have also seen some of these patients misdiagnosed as "piriformis syndrome".

Electronic Supplementary Material The online version of this chapter https://doi.org/10.1007/978-3-319-71943-6_12. contains supplementary material, which is available to authorized users.

G. Tender (✉)
Louisiana State University, New Orleans, LA, USA

A. Waguespack
Spinecare Medical Group, Marrero, LA, USA

C. Crutcher • A. Digiorgio
Department of Neurosurgery, Louisiana State University Health Sciences Center, New Orleans, LA, USA
e-mail: ccrutc@lsuhsc.edu; Adigi2@lsuhsc.edu

R. Nader
Texas Center for Neurosciences PLLC, Houston, TX, USA

American Board of Neurological Surgery, Chicago, IL, USA

Division of Neurosurgery, University of Texas Medical Branch, Galveston, TX, USA

William Carey University, Hattiesburg, MS, USA

Department of Neurosurgery, Tulane University, New Orleans, LA, USA

G. Tender (ed.), *Minimally Invasive Spine Surgery Techniques*,
https://doi.org/10.1007/978-3-319-71943-6_12

Indications

The SI joint fusion is indicated if there is sufficient evidence that the joint is a primary pain generator. NASS has specific guidelines that should be fulfilled in order for the patient to be considered a candidate for the SI joint fusion.

Symptoms: The patient typically has unilateral pain that is caudal to the lumbar spine (L5 vertebrae), localized over the posterior SIJ, and consistent with SIJ pain. The patient should NOT have generalized pain behavior (e.g. somatoform disorder) or generalized pain disorders (e.g. fibromyalgia).

Physical examination: The patient should have localized tenderness with palpation over the sacral sulcus (Fortin's point, at the insertion of the long dorsal ligament inferior to the posterior superior iliac spine or PSIS) in the absence of tenderness of similar severity elsewhere (e.g. greater trochanter, lumbar spine, coccyx). The patient should have positive response to at least 3 provocative tests (e.g. thigh thrust test, compression test, Gaenslen's test, distraction test, Patrick's sign, posterior provocation test).

Diagnostic imaging: Studies have not been shown to reliably predict pain arising from the SI joint, but are sometimes necessary to identify other pathologic conditions that may be the source of the patient's back pain:

- Plain radiographs and a CT or MRI of the SI joint should exclude the presence of destructive lesions (e.g. tumor, infection) or inflammatory arthropathy that would not be properly addressed by percutaneous SIJ fusion. Occasionally, the imaging may show evidence of SI joint injury and/or degeneration, although imaging studies have not been shown to reliably predict SI joint pain.
- Pelvis AP plain radiograph should rule out concomitant hip pathology
- Imaging of the lumbar spine (CT or MRI) should rule out neural compression or other degenerative conditions that can be causing low back or buttock pain

Treatment: The patient should have undergone and failed a minimum 6 months of intensive non-operative treatment, that must include medication optimization, activity modification, bracing, and active therapeutic exercise targeted at the lumbar spine, pelvis, SIJ, and hip, including a home exercise program.

Response to SI joint injections: The patient should have at least 75% reduction of pain for the expected duration of the anesthetic used following an image-guided, contrast-enhanced intra-articular SIJ injection on two separate occasions.

According to the ISASS guidelines, the patient should have the following documentation:

- A complete history and physical documenting the likely existence of SI joint pain;
- Performance of a fluoroscopically- guided SI joint block on the affected side (or both sides, see discussion above) which shows at least a 75% acute reduction in pain;
- A course of conservative treatment to include use of non-steroidal anti-inflammatory drugs and/or opioids (unless contraindicated) and one of the following: (1) an adequate period of rest, (2) an adequate course of physical therapy wherein the physical therapist specifically documents lack of response to treatment, (3) SI joint steroid injections into the affected joint with inadequate

response or return of pain after weeks to months, or (4) radiofrequency ablation of the affected SI joint with either inadequate response or return of pain after weeks to months;
- SI joint pain has continued for a minimum of 6 months;
- All other diagnoses that could be causing the patient's pain have been ruled out.

Contraindications

- Any case that does not fulfill ALL of the above criteria
- Presence of systematic arthropathy such as ankylosing spondylitis or rheumatoid arthritis
- Presence of generalized pain behavior (e.g., somatoform disorder) or generalized pain disorder (e.g., fibromyalgia)
- Presence of infection, tumor, or fracture
- Presence of acute, traumatic instability of the SIJ
- Presence of neural compression, as seen on an MRI or CT, that correlates with the patient's symptoms, or another, more likely, source for the pain.

Surgical Technique

There are many spine companies offering a plethora of design implants, each of them with potential advantages over the original design (e.g., graft window, compression against the joint etc). However, the surgical technique is similar and based on anatomic landmarks rather than implant design. Below we describe the originally described surgical technique, with triangular shape implants.

Patient Positioning

The patient is placed on the operative table in prone position, with the arms tucked to the sides and adequate padding for all pressure points. We prefer to use a Jackson table, in order to allow free movement of the C-arm under the patient's pelvis. Regardless of the table used, it is important for the patient's lumbar spine, pelvis, and hips to be in neutral position (i.e., not in flexion or extension).

First, we make sure the patient is in true prone position. We take an AP image and adjust the table, not the C-arm, until the spinous process of L5 is perfectly centered between the two pedicles.

On lateral fluoroscopy, the true sacral orientation is obtained by holding a straight instrument (e.g., the long blunt guide pin) perfectly vertical ("plumb line"), next to the patient, and then turning the image on the monitor until the instrument image is vertical.

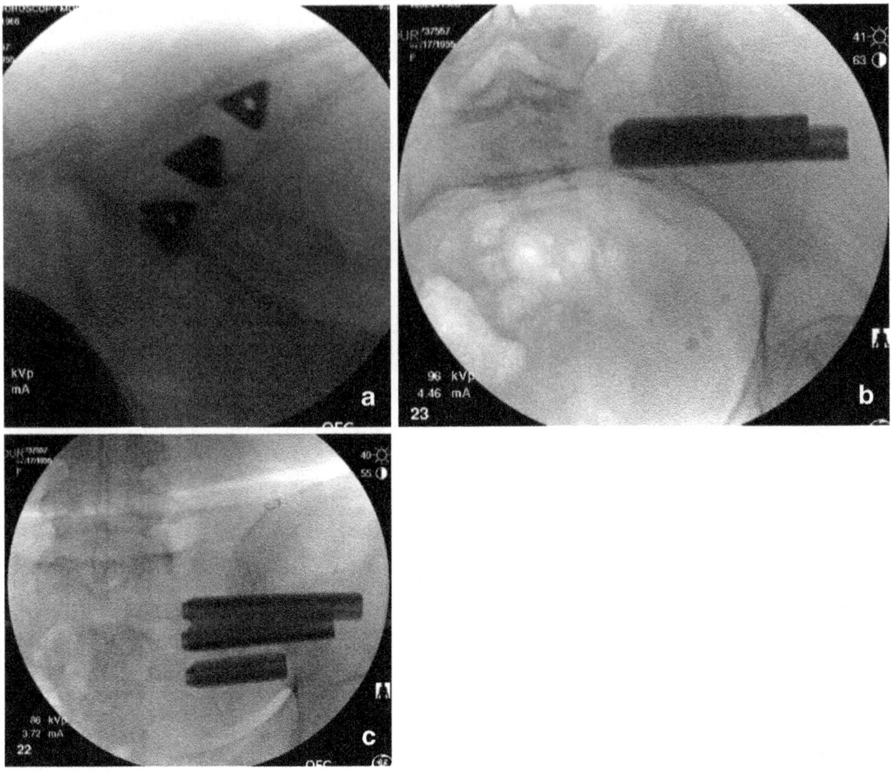

Fig. 12.1 The typical views confirming the good placement of the instrumentation after an SI joint fusion: (**a**) lateral, (**b**) inlet, and (**c**) outlet

The perfect lateral image is then obtained by wagging the C-arm until the two alar lines are superimposed. At this time, the iliac crests should also overlap and the S1 endplate should appear as a single line.

The radiology technician is advised at the beginning of the case regarding the 3 specific positions needed during the case: the lateral view, the inlet view, and the outlet view (Fig. 12.1).

The inlet view is obtained with the C-arm angled caudally about 20° from the AP view, until the S1 and S2 dense anterior cortex lines overlap. As the name suggests, the inlet view shows the pelvic inlet very well.

The outlet view is obtained with the C-arm angled cranially about 30° from the AP view, until the S1 and S2 sacral foramina can be clearly identified.

The outlet oblique view is an "enhanced" version of the outlet view, obtained by "rotating the C" of the C-arm about 15° away from the operative side and centering it on the SIJ of interest. This view is in line with the SIJ and allows for the best visualization of the targeted SIJ and the ipsilateral neuroforamina.

All these views are marked on the floor and on the C-arm, to allow the radiology technician to switch flawlessly between them.

Marks are then made on the skin in line with the underlying osseous landmarks, using the blunt guide pin. The alar line and then a longitudinal line marking the center of the sacral body are drawn on the patient.

Skin Incision and Pin Insertion

The side of the lateral pelvis and the buttock are prepped and draped in the usual sterile fashion. After infiltration with local anesthetic, a 3 cm skin incision is made with the 10-blade in line with the mark overlying the center of the sacrum, starting 1 cm caudal to the mark overlying the sacral alar line.

Under lateral fluoroscopic imaging, a guide pin is centered halfway between the anterior cortex of the sacrum and the anterior border of the spinal canal, 1 cm distal to the alar line. The pin is then impacted gently to engage the lateral cortex of the ilium.

The C-arm is then repositioned to the inlet view, under which the trajectory of the pin is adjusted so that the pin is aiming for the middle third of the S1 vertebral body. The pin adjustments should be made in a plane parallel to the surface of the C-arm receiver. Once the trajectory is considered optimal, the pin is advanced until the tip engages into the SIJ.

The C-arm is then repositioned to the outlet view, under which the trajectory of the pin is adjusted to stay parallel to the S1 endplate. This trajectory should project just cranial to the S1 foramen in the outlet view. The pin is then advanced to the desired depth under fluoroscopic guidance in the outlet view, typically a few mm lateral to the lateral aspect of the foramen. Final pin position is confirmed in both the outlet and inlet views.

Insertion of the First Implant

The soft tissue dissector is then placed into the wound over the pin, in the direction of the muscle fibers, down to the level of the lateral iliac bone, and then rotated circumferentially to dissect the muscle. The soft tissue protector with the pin sleeve in place is then inserted over the pin, down to the level of the iliac bone. The depth gauge is then used to determine the appropriate implant length.

The pin sleeve is the removed and the high-speed drill is placed advanced over the pin, under the outlet view, to a point just medial to the SI joint, through the lateral sacral cortex and avoiding the sacral foramina. Care is taken to keep the drill collinear to the pin, since any difference in direction may push the sharp pin into the foramen and potentially cause nerve damage. The drill is then removed under power, using the exchange pin to maintain the original sharp pin in place. Using the soft tissue protector, the triangular broach is then oriented under lateral fluoroscopy so that one of its' surfaces is parallel to the alar line. The C-arm is changed back to the outlet view and the broach is advanced through the SIJ, until two of its teeth are engaged into the sacrum. The broach is then removed, leaving the pin in place. The first iFuse implant is then placed over the pin, bullet nose towards the patient, utilizing the outlet view to confirm depth and trajectory, and leaving the implant about 2 mm lateral to the sacral foramen. Final imaging in all 3 views (inlet, outlet, and lateral) confirms the adequate placement of the implant (Fig. 12.1).

Insertion of the Second and Third Implants

The 15 mm fixed parallel pin guide is then utilized to position the second pin. The short tube of the pin guide is placed over the existing pin and advanced until it hits the iliac bone. Under lateral fluoroscopy, the guide is then rotated until the tip of the long tube is at the anterior sacral line. The second pin is then inserted through the long tube and its tip is engaged into the cortical bone of the ilium. The pin is advanced and then the second implant is inserted in a similar fashion as the first one.

The same steps are repeated for the insertion of the third implant. Final imaging in all 3 views should show good placement of the 3 implants.

Closure

After this, the wound is irrigated with antibiotic solution and the gluteal muscles are injected with Exparel for postoperative pain control. The would is closed in layers with interrupted 2-0 Vycril on a UR needle for the gluteal fascia, followed by 3-0 Vycril and running subcutaneous 4-0 Monocryl for the skin.

Tricks and Pitfalls

This surgical technique is relatively straightforward and with a low rate of complications.

Once the drill is used and cancellous bone is exposed, brisk bleeding is expected, until the implant is impacted. Therefore, the surgeon should proceed with a sense of urgency during these steps.

The most common mistake is to inadvertently advance the guide pin into the S1 foramen with either the drill or the broach, if the two are not perfectly aligned, particularly during the insertion of the second implant. We recommend exchanging the sharp guide pin with a blunt one, before starting drilling, so that no nerve injury can be expected, even if the guide pin inadvertently enters the foramen.

Placement of the three implants allows for some variability regarding their position. The SI joint extends anteriorly over a distance, but this can only be visualized during an arthrogram, not during surgery on the usual lateral fluoroscopic images. Some surgeons place the second implant anterior to the anterior sacral line, knowing the approximate position of the SI joint. We prefer to stay close to the anterior sacral line when inserting the second implant.

Complications

Since this is a relatively new procedure, the complications may be underreported in the literature.

The most common complication is probably the S1 nerve injury, due to inadvertent violation of the respective foramen by either the guide pin or, less likely, the drill/broach/implant. Avoidance of this complication involves use of a blunt guide pin and frequent usage of the outlet view imaging when drilling and broaching.

Pseudarthrosis after this procedure is evidenced by persistence of recurrence of symptoms and lucency around the implants on the CT scan. Revision surgery can be performed through the same minimally invasive incision and involves removal of the original implants, if possible, followed by insertion of new, threaded, implants, via new created trajectories [1, 2].

Vascular injuries with this approach [3] are rare and can be avoided by using the proper surgical technique and imaging.

Literature Review

This relatively new procedure has been relatively well received by the surgical community. Probably one of the reasons is that, once SI joint has been recognized as a source of pain, we have been able to treat many of these patients with intractable low back pain and no spinal pathology [4–6]. Another reason is that adequately diagnosed patients tend to do very well after the minimally invasive surgical fusion, as opposed to the conservative treatment [7–14]. The reported complications are rare, but can be potentially serious [3].

Conclusions

The minimally invasive sacro-iliac joint fusion has excellent results in the properly diagnosed patients and has relatively low morbidity.

References

1. Spain K, Holt T. Surgical revision after sacroiliac joint fixation or fusion. Int J Spine Surg. 2017;11:5. https://doi.org/10.14444/4005.
2. MenMuir B, Fielding LC. Revision of minimally invasive sacroiliac joint fixation: technical considerations and case studies using decortication and threaded implant fixation. Int J Spine Surg. 2017;11:8. https://doi.org/10.14444/4008.
3. Palmiere C, Augsburger M, Del Mar Lesta M, Grabherr S, Borens O. Fatal hemorrhage following sacroiliac joint fusion surgery: a case report. Leg Med. 2017;26:102–5. https://doi.org/10.1016/j.legalmed.2015.06.006.
4. Rashbaum RF, Ohnmeiss DD, Lindley EM, Kitchel SH, Patel VV. Sacroiliac joint pain and its treatment. Clin Spine Surg. 2016;29:42–8. https://doi.org/10.1097/bsd.0000000000000359.
5. Cher D, Polly D, Berven S. Sacroiliac joint pain: burden of disease. Med Devices. 2014; 7:73–81. https://doi.org/10.2147/mder.s59437.
6. Shaffrey CI, Smith JS. Stabilization of the sacroiliac joint. Neurosurg Focus. 2013;35, Editorial. https://doi.org/10.3171/2013.v2.focus13273.
7. Vanaclocha V, Herrera JM, Saiz-Sapena N, Rivera-Paz M, Verdu-Lopez F. Minimally invasive sacroiliac joint fusion, radiofrequency denervation, and conservative management for sacroiliac joint pain: 6-year comparative case series. Neurosurgery. 2017. https://doi.org/10.1093/neuros/nyx185.
8. Sturesson B, et al. Six-month outcomes from a randomized controlled trial of minimally invasive SI joint fusion with triangular titanium implants vs conservative management. Eur Spine J. 2017;26:708–19. https://doi.org/10.1007/s00586-016-4599-9.
9. Kancherla VK, McGowan SM, Audley BN, Sokunbi G, Puccio ST. Patient reported outcomes from sacroiliac joint fusion. Asian Spine J. 2017;11:120–6. https://doi.org/10.4184/asj.2017.11.1.120.
10. Dengler J, et al. Predictors of outcome in conservative and minimally invasive surgical management of pain originating from the sacroiliac joint: a pooled analysis. Spine. 2017;42:1664. https://doi.org/10.1097/brs.0000000000002169.
11. Bornemann R, et al. Two-year clinical results of patients with sacroiliac joint syndrome treated by arthrodesis using a triangular implant system. Technol Health Care. 2017;25:319–25. https://doi.org/10.3233/thc-161272.
12. Sachs D, et al. Durable intermediate-to long-term outcomes after minimally invasive transiliac sacroiliac joint fusion using triangular titanium implants. Med Devices. 2016;9:213–22. https://doi.org/10.2147/mder.s109276.
13. Saavoss JD, Koenig L, Cher DJ. Productivity benefits of minimally invasive surgery in patients with chronic sacroiliac joint dysfunction. Clinicoecon Outcomes Res. 2016;8:77–85. https://doi.org/10.2147/ceor.s101607.
14. Polly DW, et al. Two-year outcomes from a randomized controlled trial of minimally invasive sacroiliac joint fusion vs. non-surgical management for sacroiliac joint dysfunction. Int J Spine Surg. 2016;10:28. https://doi.org/10.14444/3028.

Chapter 13
Lumbar Retroperitoneal Transpsoas Corpectomy

Gabriel Tender, Durga R. Sure, Yasser Badr, Anthony Digiorgio, and Clifford Crutcher

Introduction

The standard surgical treatment for lumbar corpectomy is usually performed by the spine surgeon with the assistance of the general surgeon and involves extensive abdominal wall dissection and psoas muscle mobilization. Thoracic and lumbar corpectomies can be performed via a posterior or postero-lateral approach [1–3] or an antero-lateral (transthoracic/retroperitoneal) approach [4, 5]. The minimally invasive surgery (MIS) option for the lateral approach has been successfully used in the thoracic spine (T5–L1) with good results [4, 5], since the dissection for exposing these levels is extrapleural. However, this approach becomes more difficult in the lower lumbar spine, and particularly at L4, due to the presence of the psoas muscle and the enclosed lumbar plexus. We describe the minimally invasive lateral retroperitoneal technique, in which the psoas muscle is dissected rather than mobilized.

Electronic Supplementary Material The online version of this chapter https://doi.org/10.1007/978-3-319-71943-6_13. contains supplementary material, which is available to authorized users.

G. Tender (✉)
Louisiana State University, New Orleans, LA, USA

D.R. Sure
Essentia Health, Duluth, MN, USA

Y. Badr
Badr Brain and Spine, Los Angeles, CA, USA

A. Digiorgio • C. Crutcher
Department of Neurosurgery, Louisiana State University Health Sciences Center, New Orleans, LA, USA
e-mail: Adigi2@lsuhsc.edu; ccrutc@lsuhsc.edu

G. Tender (ed.), *Minimally Invasive Spine Surgery Techniques*,
https://doi.org/10.1007/978-3-319-71943-6_13

Indications

The minimally invasive lateral retroperitoneal approach can be performed for L1 through L4 corpectomy. The lesions affecting the vertebral body that needs to be resected can be traumatic, tumoral, or infectious.

Trauma

The classification and indications for surgical treatment in thoracolumbar fractures have evolved over the past 50 years along with the diagnostic capabilities. Currently, the thoracolumbar injury classification and severity (TLICS) system takes into account fracture morphology, posterior ligamentous complex (PLC) integrity, and neurological status [6, 7]. In patients with comminuted vertebral body fractures and posterior ligamentous complex disruption, a circumferential (anterior and posterior) fixation is recommended.

Tumors

Primary or metastatic tumors can affect the lumbar vertebral bodies and may result in either loss of vertebral body height with kyphotic deformity and/or anterior cauda equina and/or conus medullaris compression. These tumors can be successfully approached via the minimally invasive lateral retroperitoneal approach. However, if the tumor extends into the pedicles and/or has a significant component in the lateral or posterior spinal canal, the postero-lateral approach may provide better circumferential decompression of the canal.

Infection

In cases of discitis, the minimally invasive lateral retroperitoneal approach offers an excellent route to perform an extensive disc debridement and possibly decompression of an anterior epidural abscess compressing the spinal sac. We prefer not to use instrumentation in these cases until the infection is controlled. However, occasionally, there is extensive destruction of the adjacent vertebral bodies and major neurological deficits due to compression of the cauda equina and/or conus medullaris. Almost invariably, these patients also present with significant kyphotic deformity. In this situation, a 2-level corpectomy with decompression of the spinal canal and reconstruction with an expandable cage may become mandatory.

Contraindications

The L5 vertebral body and the L5–S1 disc cannot be accessed via the transpsoas approach.

The L4 corpectomy feasibility depends on the L4–5 disc level anatomy. If the femoral nerve is anteriorly located (as seen on the T2-weighted axial MRI) or if the iliac crests project above the L4 mid-body on the lateral X-ray, then a different approach may be indicated.

Retroperitoneal scarring represents a relative contraindication.

Preoperative Planning

Preoperative imaging includes:

1. MRI: shows the position of the femoral nerve (on the T2-weighted axial images) and the status of the posterior ligamentous complex (on STIR images);
2. Lateral and AP X-rays: show the relative height of the iliac crests and the local deformity;
3. CT: shows the morphology of the fracture and possibly abnormal bony anatomy.

Surgical Technique

Shallow Docking

The patient is placed in lateral decubitus (preferably right, but it depends on whether there is coronal deformity) and taped to the operating table in a fashion similar to the lateral transpsoas discectomy technique, previously described in Chap. 7 as well as the literature [8]. Patients' true lateral position is verified by fluoroscopy [9]. The targeted vertebral body is marked on the skin, based on the lateral fluoroscopic image, and a 6–8 cm skin incision is centered on the targeted segment, parallel to the iliac crest (for L3 and L4) or over the corresponding rib (for L1 and L2). The incision is carried down through the superficial muscle fascia and then the underlying muscles (major oblique, minor oblique, and transversalis) are bluntly dissected until the retroperitoneal fat is accessed. The opening in the lateral abdominal wall muscles is enlarged enough to accommodate a retractor spanning the space between the discs above and below the targeted vertebral body. We recommend bluntly dissecting each muscle layer separately and over a distance of about 8–10 cm (retracting the skin in both directions to do it), with care to protect any nerve encountered (the ilioinguinal and iliohypogastric nerves run parallel to the iliac crest in between the muscle layers). The exposed retroperitoneal fat is gently separated from the posterior wall under direct visualization (the lateral femoral cutaneous nerve runs on the anterior aspect of the transversalis fascia) until the transverse processes and the psoas muscle anterior to them is encountered. A superficial retractor is then placed on the surface of the psoas and attached to the side of the table with the appropriate rigid arm. The rest of the technique is different for each level and will be described individually.

L4

The L4 corpectomy is the most challenging one, because the femoral nerve can occasionally be located more anteriorly at the L4–5 disc level and the iliac crest can make the access to the L4–5 disc more difficult, particularly in males.

The L4–5 discectomy is performed first, using the transpsoas technique previously described in Chap. 7 as well as the literature [8]. If the discectomy cannot be done safely, the procedure can be aborted without having destabilized the L3–4 level. We prefer the direct visualization technique, but the EMG-based technique can also be used. The location of the discectomy is chosen keeping in mind that the exposed L5 endplate will be supporting the caudal footplate of the expandable cage; thus, if more lordosis is desired, a more anterior position for the discectomy is selected. Then, the retractor is removed and re-inserted at the L3–4 level, and the procedure is repeated for the L3–4 discectomy (Video 13.1). The final repositioning is started with the retractor inserted through the psoas at L4–5 and then gently opened cranially, while holding downward pressure, to separate the muscle fibers longitudinally, until the L3–4 discectomy site is encountered. The cranial and caudal blades of the retractor are centered at the previously performed discectomy sites, whereas the posterior blade is placed about 1 cm anterior to the dorsal border of L4 on the lateral fluoroscopic image, in order to protect the dorsal-running femoral nerve. A fourth, fan-like retractor is added anteriorly to keep the retroperitoneal organs and the anterior psoas fibers separated from the operative field.

An alternative to this part of the procedure is to start the psoas dissection at the level of the L4 mid-vertebral body and continue cranially and caudally until the L3–4 and L4–5 discs, respectively, are encountered (Video 13.2). The obvious advantage of this variant is that the retractor does not have to be repositioned twice. The disadvantages are: (1) The psoas dissection has to be well planned, in order for the exposed L4–5 and L3–4 discs to provide optimal position for the discectomy; (2) A special self-retaining retractor is necessary, with blades that are wide enough to span the distance between the L3 inferior endplate to the L5 superior endplate (this retractor is not part of the routine instrumentation set).

At this time, a neuromonitoring ball-tip probe, as well as direct operative microscope visualization, can be used to confirm that the femoral nerve is not exposed in the operative field. After coagulating and cutting the segmental vessels, an L4 corpectomy is then performed between the two discectomy sites, with enough bone removal to easily accommodate the expandable cage, in order to minimize the risk of cage insertion pushing any bone fragments posteriorly into the spinal canal. The corpectomy has to be done relatively fast, since the exposed cancellous bone can result in significant blood loss, particularly if the corpectomy is done for a metastasis from a vascular tumor (e.g., renal cell carcinoma). Therefore, we often use osteotomes for this part of the procedure, with the posterior cut placed roughly at the junction between the anterior two thirds and the posterior third of the vertebral body (this eliminates the risk of spinal canal violation). Once the height of the cage is determined, Floseal or analogues can be placed to decrease cancellous bone bleeding. The contralateral annulus fibrosus at L3–4 and L4–5 is penetrated with a sharp Cobb. Trials mimicking the cage's footplates are used to determine the appropriate length as well as to make sure the footplate will not be blocked by residual disc material near the contralateral annulus. The cage is then inserted between two sliding blades, in order to protect the endplates, and expanded under frequent AP fluoroscopic guidance. A tactile feel, as well as direct visualization, also guide the amount of expansion needed.

The next step, necessary in patients with posteriorly displaced fracture fragments or tumor, is to decompress the spinal canal. The retractor is slightly angled into an oblique anterior to posterior direction (20–30°), holding downward pressure not to lose contact between the tip of the posterior blade and the L4 vertebral body. The high-speed drill is used to thin out the fragments protruding in the spinal canal and a long, bayoneted, small-cup, straight curette is used to separate the posterior longitudinal ligament from the lumbar dura mater and push the ligament along with the remainder of the fractured fragments anteriorly, away from the spinal canal. It is important to custom order this instrument (the long, bayoneted, small-cup, straight curette) since it does not come in any of the regular sets. Copious bleeding from the lumbar epidural venous plexus usually occurs and can be controlled with gelatin thrombin hemostatic sealants and gentle pressure. The decompression is continued in the cranial and caudal direction until the respective discs are encountered, as well as towards the contralateral side, until the level of the contralateral pedicle is reached, on the AP fluoroscopic image. Once the decompression is completed, the dura mater of the spinal sac typically expands into the operative field, back into its' normal anatomic position. After careful hemostasis, the retractor is removed and the wound is closed in layers over a Jackson-Pratt drain.

L3

The L3 corpectomy is usually easier than L4, since the iliac crest height is almost never an issue and the femoral nerve is typically posteriorly located (Video 13.4). Moreover, the exposure is below the rib cage and therefore no rib resection is necessary. The kidney may appear to be in the way on MRI axial images, but typically it mobilizes easily anteriorly. At this level, the psoas muscle is thinner and allows for easier dissection compared to L4.

L2

The L2 corpectomy is still retroperitoneal, although the diaphragm insertion on the underside of the rib is often encountered. After partially removing the overlying rib (the tip of the eleventh rib, typically), we recommend penetrating the diaphragm superficially, under the rib, rather than in the depth, next to the vertebral body. The psoas muscle is thin and easy to dissect.

L1

The L1 corpectomy is actually approached in a retropleural, rather than retroperitoneal, fashion (Video 13.3). After partially removing the overlying rib (the tenth rib, typically), the parietal pleura is encountered. Blunt finger dissection allows detachment of the parietal pleura from the remainder of the tenth rib, as well as the ninth and eleventh intact ribs. Following the ribs proximally, the finger (or a Kittner dissector) eventually encounters the junction with the vertebral body. We try to protect the parietal pleura integrity as much as possible, as it serves as a barrier between the retractor blades and the lung; however, in the depth, the parietal pleura is often adherent to the vertebral body and, upon placement of the retractor, the intrapleural space is exposed, with the tip of the lung often seen coming in and out of the field with each breath (there is no need for dual-lumen intubation and lung deflation). The retractor is placed over the fractured vertebral body (on lateral fluoroscopy), which requires some anterior and downward pressure against the diaphragm. Once the retractor is locked in place, the microscope is brought into the operative field.

The first structure exposed is the diaphragm's insertion on the L1 vertebral body. This can be sharply transected and then closed at the end of the operation, although we have left it open numerous times without any postoperative complications. The next layer is the very thin psoas muscle, which can be detached with the Bovie cautery, but with care to preserve the segmental vessels (the artery must be tested, before transection, to make sure Adamkiewicz artery does not originate at this level).

Pearls and Pitfalls

Positioning

Taping the patient to the table is similar to the LLIF technique. For a perfect lateral image, we usually place the patient in slight Trendelenburg.

After taping, we first get an AP image, to confirm that the patient is in perfect lateral decubitus. The table, not the C-arm, is tilted left or right until the spinous process of the level of interest is perfectly centered between the pedicles on the AP image. The C-arm is then used to draw on the skin the projection of the vertebral body of interest.

Exposure

As mentioned, the muscle layers must be divided bluntly over about 10 cm, as they have different directions and must accommodate a wider exposure than the one for a simple lateral discectomy. At L1 and L2, part of the overlying rib must be resected to achieve the exposure.

While the psoas muscle runs obliquely in a cranial to caudal and posterior to anterior direction, the muscle fibers direction is not exactly parallel to the desired cage direction. Since it is easier to retract the muscle fibers anteriorly, we prefer to dissect the muscle fibers more posterior over the caudal disc, if possible, and retract the psoas fibers anteriorly over the cranial disc.

Discectomy and Endplate Preparation

Since the discs have a bi-convex shape (unless severely degenerated, in which case they become flat), endplate preparation must be done respecting its' concave shape. The best preparation, in our opinion, is done with a wide Cobb (20 or 22 mm) that follows the dissection plane between the disc and the endplate. As the Cobb follows the concave surface of the endplate, the direction of the shaft changes from cranially angled (initially) to straight (as the tip of the Cobb passes the midpoint of the disc). If this direction is not changed, there is a risk of endplate and vertebral body violation in the deep (contralateral) half of the vertebral body.

Corpectomy

The corpectomy has to be wide enough to easily accommodate the core of the cage, so that no fragments get pushed posteriorly in the spinal canal. We typically leave a thin layer of bone in the contralateral aspect of the resected vertebral body, since that will not interfere with cage placement and at the same time will minimize morbidity from the contralateral psoas muscle.

The corpectomy also has to be done fast, since the cancellous bone (or tumoral bone) can bleed briskly at this time. For that reason, we use osteotomes to remove most of the bone, safely away from the spinal canal, and only use the high-speed drill for the second part of the osteotomy, when decompressing the spinal canal (if necessary), *after* cage insertion.

Bleeding from the cancellous (or tumoral) bone can be controlled with Floseal, which can be left in place while the endplates undergo the final preparation and the footplates are sized.

Complications

Neuro-Vascular Injury

The nerves and vessels at risk are the same as for the lateral lumbar interbody fusion technique, described in Chap. 7.

Additionally, care must be exercised before transecting the segmental vessels, particularly at the higher levels, in order to ensure that the Adamkiewicz artery does not originate from that segmental artery. We recommend temporary soft occlusion of the exposed segmental artery (e.g., with a Kittner), for about 10′; if no MEP changes are reported by neuromonitoring, than it should be safe to transect the vessel. It is important to use MEP, since SSEPs will not be changed in case of Adamkiewicz artery occlusion.

Dural Tears

Occasionally, a sharp fracture fragment can penetrate the posterior longitudinal ligament and the dura and, upon removal, can lead to CSF extravasation. More commonly, the surgeon inadvertently injures the dura at the time of fracture fragment removal. In either case, the dural tear is usually not amenable to direct repair. Instead, we recommend gentle tamponade with Gelfoam followed by DuraSeal, and placement of a lumbar drain for 5–7 days.

Inadequate Placement of the Cage

This should be recognized intraoperatively. Typically, the cage is either placed to far posteriorly, especially if the canal decompression is performed before cage insertion, or is placed at an oblique angle against the endplates. Either way, when recognized on the lateral fluoroscopic image, the cage can be repositioned more anteriorly or at the correct angle, respectively.

Case Examples

Patient 1

A 28-year-old man was brought to the emergency room after a 48-foot fall with multiple injuries, including brain contusions, facial and extremity fractures, and an L4 fracture. The neurological examination included right thigh and knee pain and mild knee extension weakness. The computed tomography (CT) scan showed a 3-column fracture with focal sagittal and coronal deformity (Fig. 13.1a–c), but no significant spinal canal compromise. Magnetic resonance imaging (MRI) confirmed PLC disruption (Fig. 13.1d). The TLICS score for the L4 fracture was 7 (morphology 2, PLC integrity 3, neurological status 2) with operative indication for a circumferential fixation. Preoperative planning included MRI analysis of the femoral nerve position between the L3–4 and L4–5 discs (Fig. 13.1e, f). A lateral X-ray showed the projection of the iliac crest at the level of the L4–5 disc space (Fig. 13.1g). A minimally invasive transpsoas L4 corpectomy was performed via a right-sided approach, with deformity correction and indirect right-sided decompression by usage of an expandable cage (Fig. 13.1h–j). Posterior pedicle screw/rod fixation was performed subsequently. A postoperative CT confirmed the adequate placement of the instrumentation and correction of deformity (Fig. 13.1k, l).

Patient 2

A 65-year-old man with schizophrenia was brought to the emergency room after a 32-foot fall with multiple rib, spine, and extremity fractures. The patient showed poor cooperation with the neurological examination, but complained of pain in the right leg and was able to move both legs spontaneously against gravity. The CT showed a 3-column fracture and retropulsion of the fracture fragments with an approximately 70% canal compromise (Fig. 13.2a–c). The MRI confirmed PLC disruption. The TLICS score for the L4 fracture was 7 (morphology 2, PLC integrity 3, neurological status 2) with operative indication for a circumferential fixation. Preoperative CT reconstruction showed the low iliac crest position (Fig. 13.2d) and the MRI showed the posterior femoral nerve location between the L3–4 and L4–5 discs (Fig. 13.2e, f). A minimally invasive transpsoas L4 corpectomy and fusion with expandable cage was performed via a left-sided approach (Fig. 13.2g–j), followed by decompression of the spinal canal. A posterior pedicle screw/rod fixation completed the operation.

The operative time and estimated blood loss were 180 min, 400 ml, and 300 min, 450 ml, respectively. Intraoperatively, the femoral nerve was not exposed in the operative field in either case. Neurostimulation behind the posterior blade in Patient 2 yielded responses between 2 and 5 mA, confirming the close proximity of the femoral nerve, as expected.

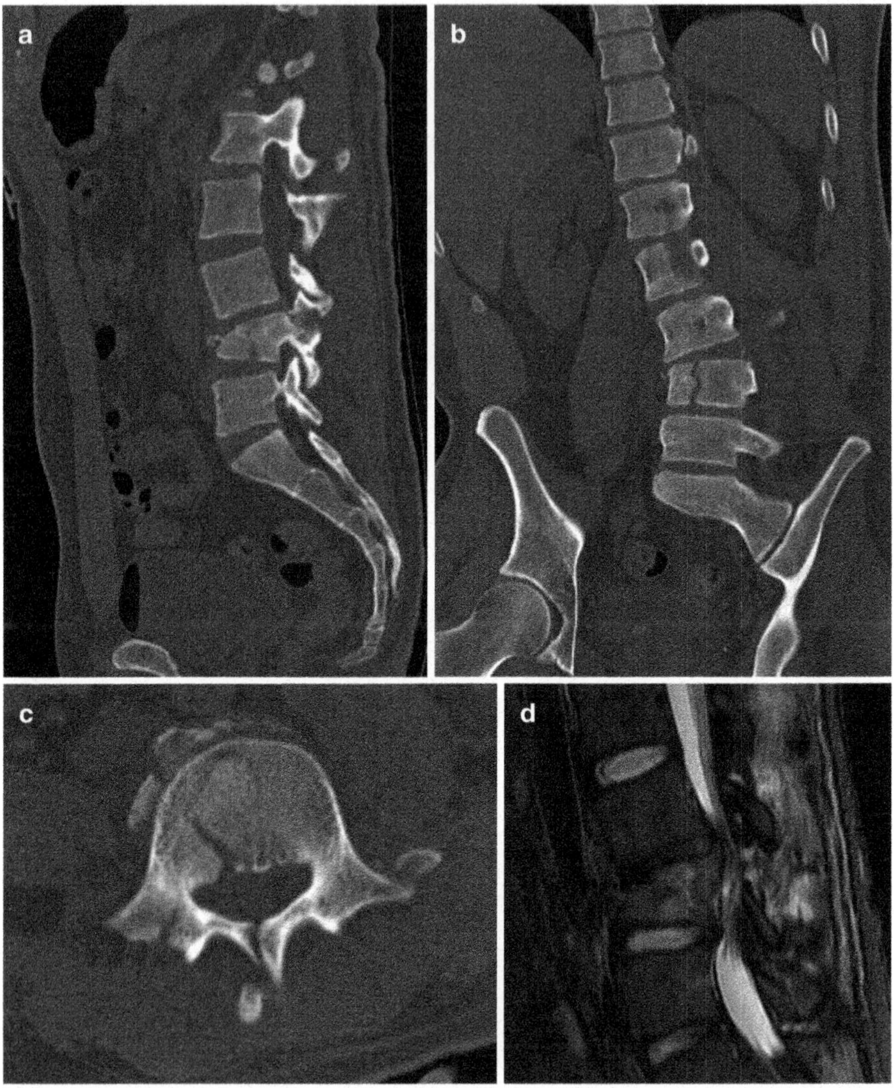

Fig. 13.1 Imaging of Patient 1. (**a**) Sagittal, (**b**) Coronal, and (**c**) Axial computed tomographic (CT) images demonstrating the 3-column L4 fracture without canal compromise; (**d**) Sagittal inversion-recovery magnetic resonance imaging (MRI) demonstrating edema in the posterior ligamentous complex; (**e**) L3–4 and (**f**) L4–5 coronal and axial MRI demonstrating the femoral nerve position in relationship to the vertebral body; (**g**) lateral x-ray demonstrating the iliac crest height at the level of L4–5 disc; (**h**) Lateral intraoperative x-ray demonstrating the cage position, following the sites of L3–4 and L4–5 discectomies and corresponding L4 corpectomy; (**i**) initial and (**j**) expanded cage on antero-posterior (AP) intraoperative x-ray; (**k**) sagittal and (**l**) coronal CT images of the final construct at 1-day postoperatively, showing reasonable correction of deformity

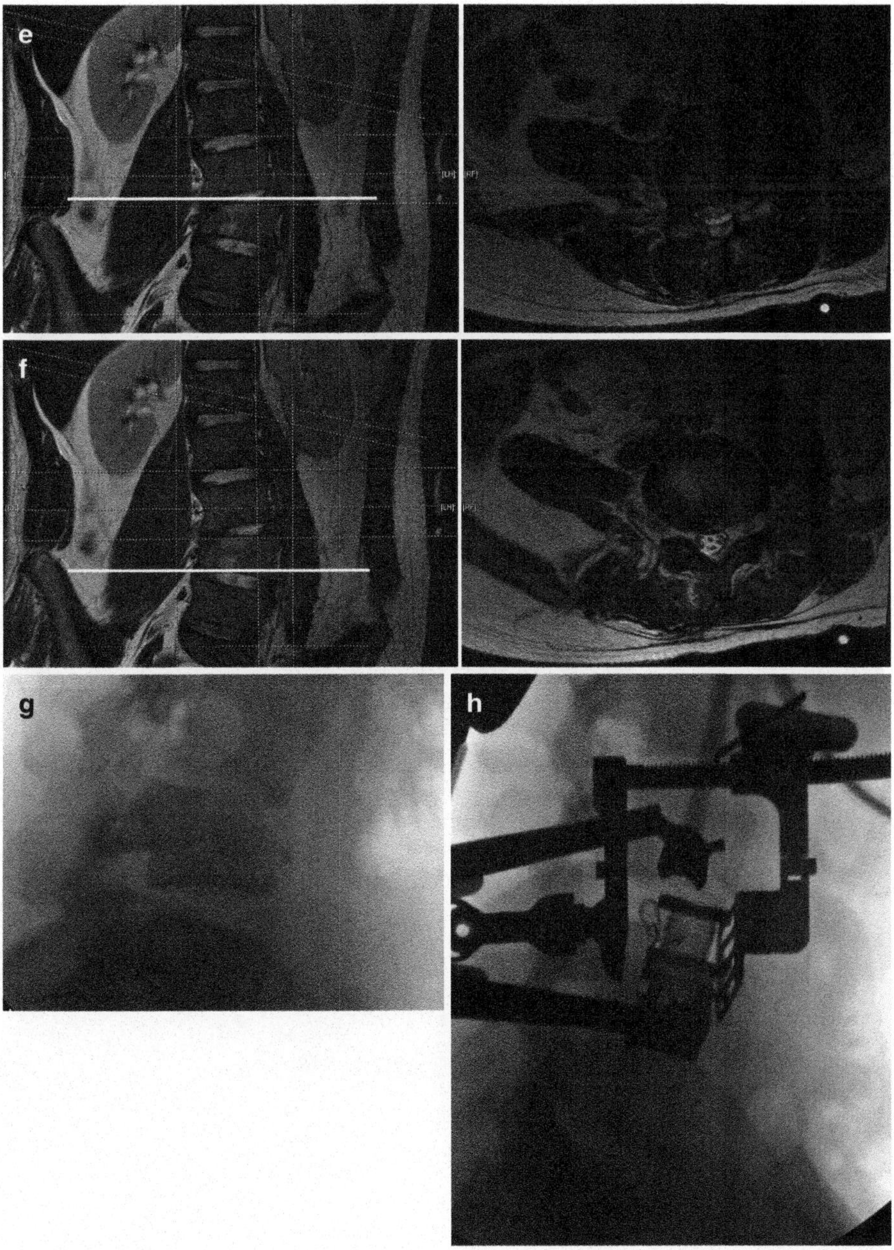

Fig. 13.1 (continued)

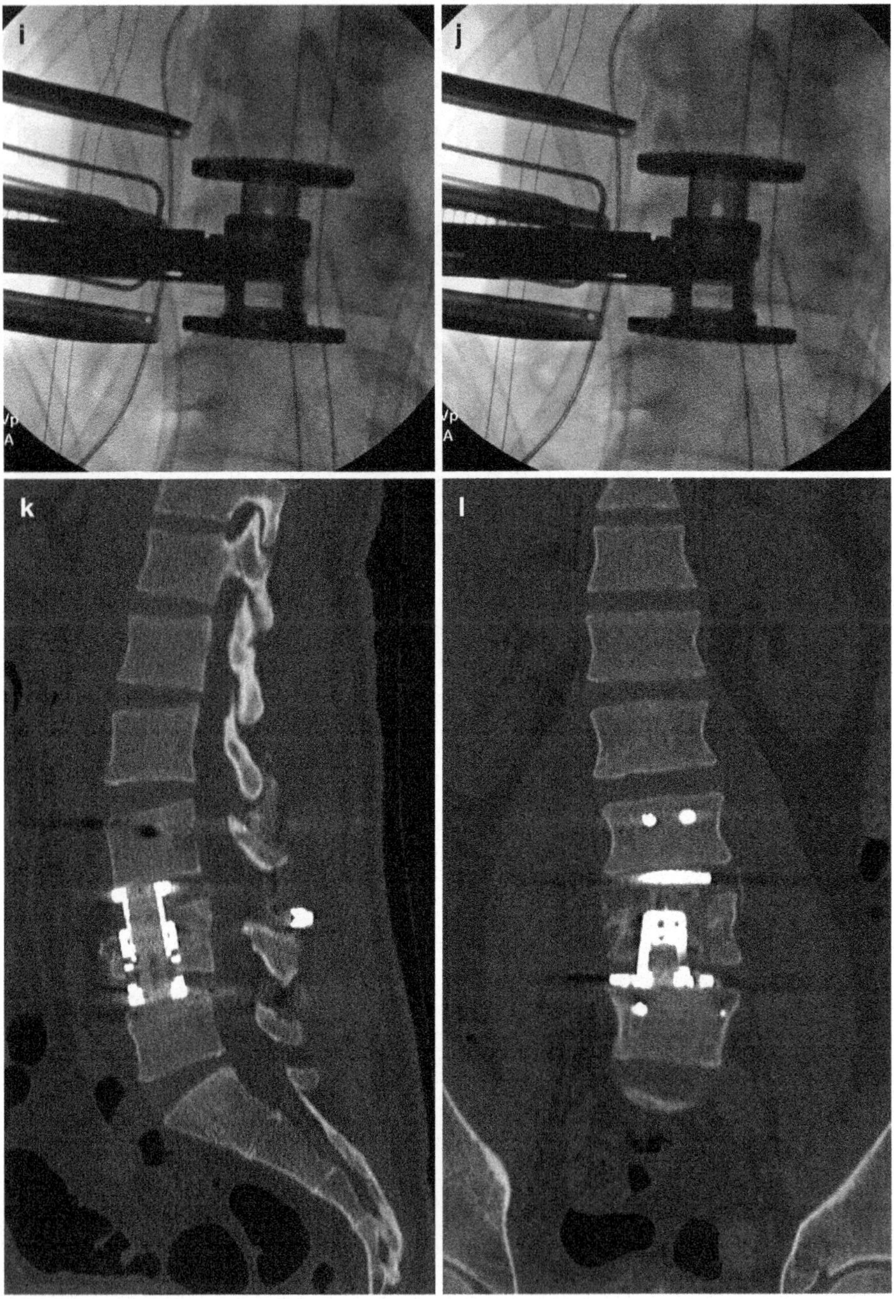

Fig. 13.1 (continued)

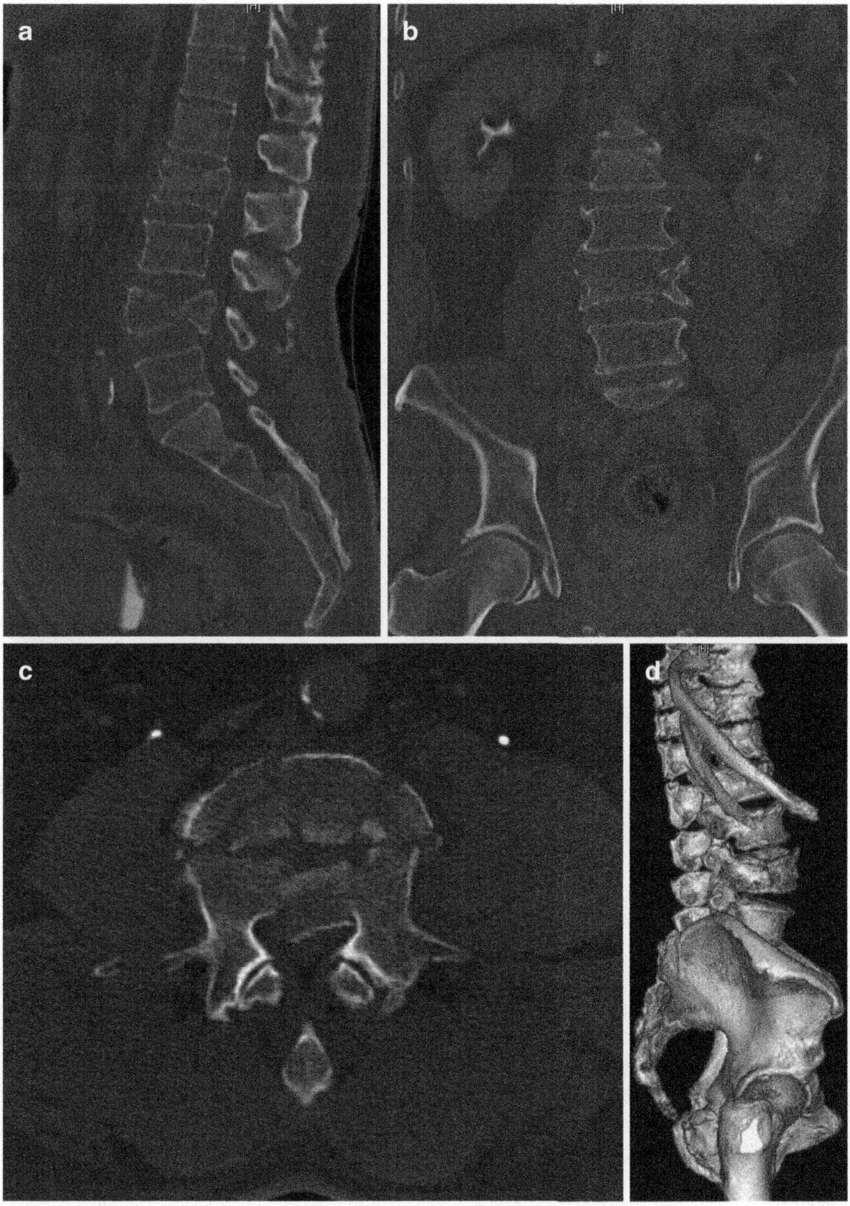

Fig. 13.2 Imaging of Patient 2. (**a**) Sagittal, (**b**) Coronal, and (**c**) Axial computed tomographic (CT) images demonstrating the 3-column L4 fracture with canal compromise; (**d**) CT reconstruction demonstrating the iliac crest height below the level of L4–5 disc; (**e**) L3–4 and (**f**) L4–5 coronal and axial magnetic resonance imaging (MRI) demonstrating the femoral nerve position in relationship to the vertebral body; (**g**) Lateral intraoperative x-ray demonstrating the retractor position, with the cranial and caudal blades following the sites of L3–4 and L4–5 discectomies, respectively, the posterior blade about 1 cm anterior to the posterior L4 vertebral body border, and the anterior fan-like retractor close to the anterior L4 border; (**h**) initial and (**i**) expanded cage on antero-posterior (AP) intraoperative x-ray; (**j**) lateral intraoperative x-ray demonstrating cage position and posterior decompression (the view is slightly oblique, to follow the direction of the posterior retractor blade)

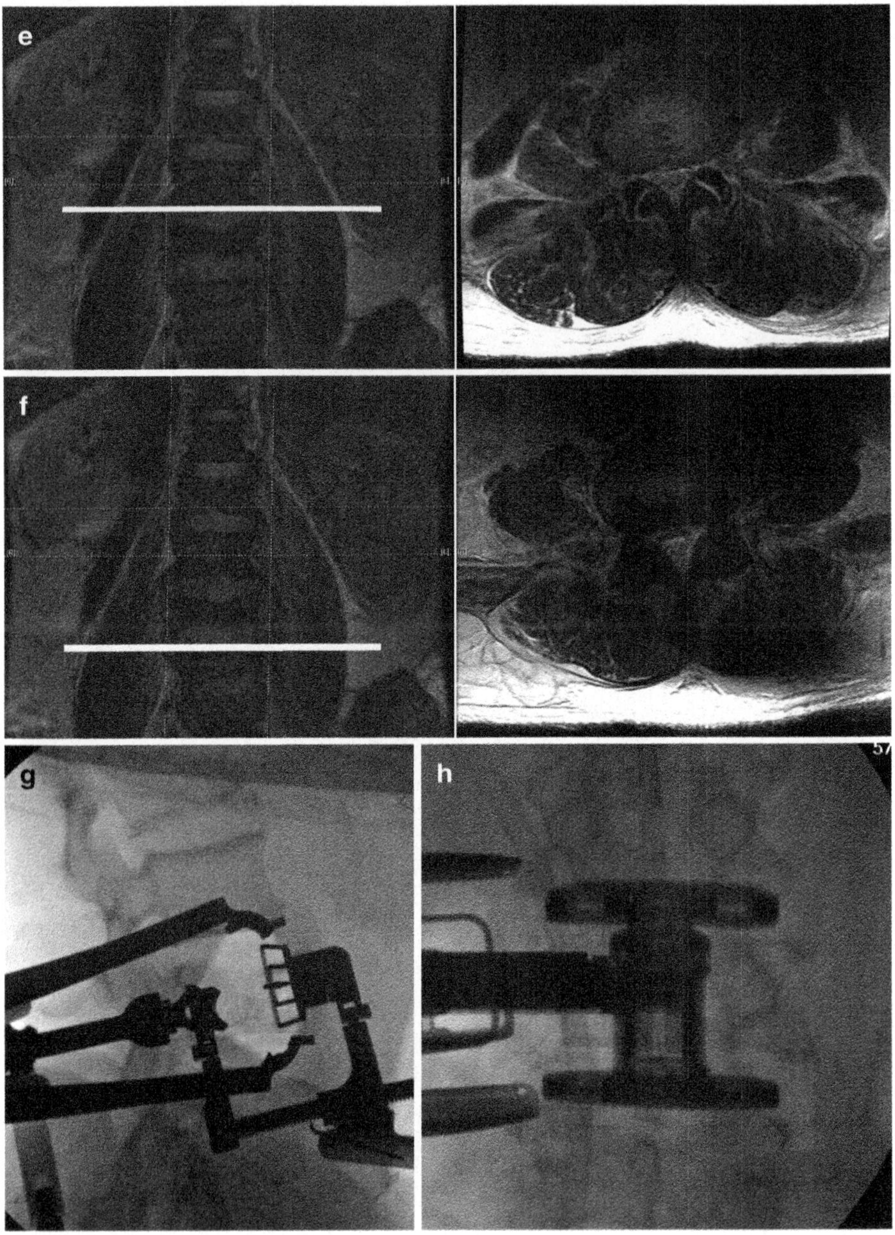

Fig. 13.2 (continued)

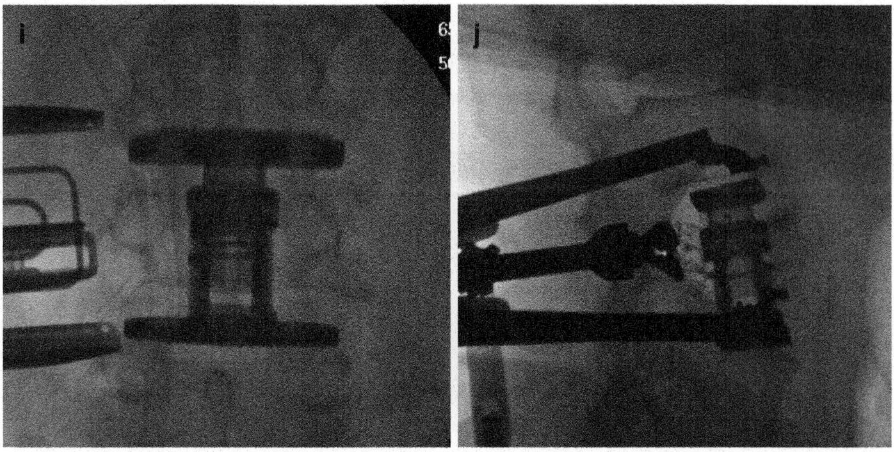

Fig. 13.2 (continued)

There were no complications related to this operation in either patient. Patient 1 exhibited pain relief in the right lower extremity at 2 weeks postoperatively and complete resolution by 6 months. Patient 2 was also mobilized immediately in a TLSO brace (due to the coexisting L2 fracture) and had no residual radicular pain. At the 6-month follow-up visit, both patients were ambulatory and with no complaints related to their lumbar fractures.

Literature Review

The lateral approach offers certain advantages compared to the posterior approaches, such as less paraspinous muscle trauma and better access angle for the spinal canal decompression, particularly with centrally located fragments [5]. The minimally invasive retropleural approach for the thoracic and upper lumbar spine has been recently described [5] and we have also used it with good results. However, in the mid-lumbar spine, and particularly at L4, the presence of the psoas muscle and the lumbar plexus has tempered the usage of a minimally invasive approach for corpectomy.

The standard open approach for L4 corpectomy is typically performed by the general surgeon and involves detachment of the psoas muscle from anterior to posterior. After psoas mobilization and corpectomy, a straight lateral exposure is required for cage insertion, especially if a wide footplate cage is desired [10]. Therefore, this type of operative technique requires a long skin incision and significant retraction of both the abdominal viscera (anteriorly) and the psoas muscle (posteriorly) (Fig. 13.3, left). The idea of a minimally invasive approach stemmed from the realization that, anatomically, the femoral nerve usually runs along the posterior

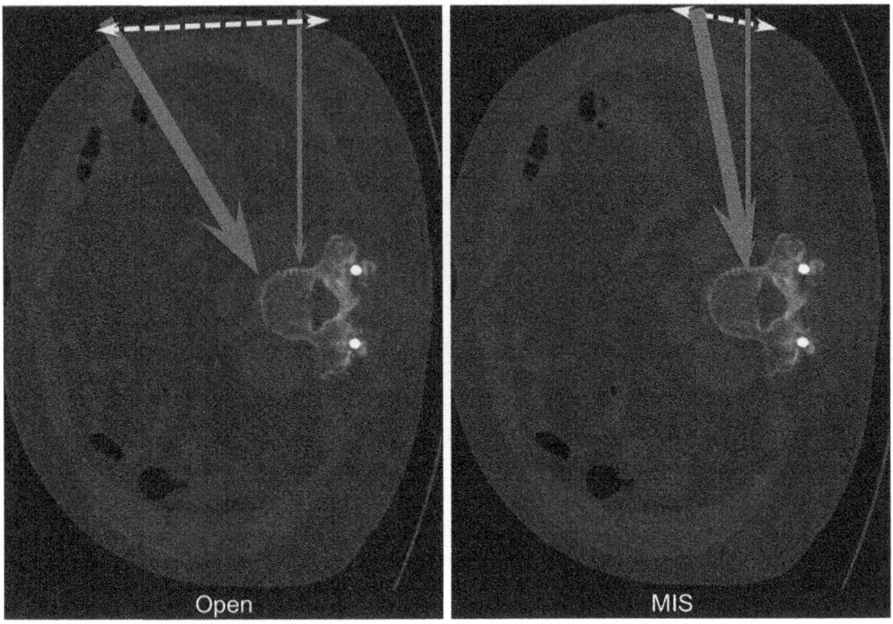

Fig. 13.3 Illustration of psoas dissection (thick arrow) and cage insertion (thin arrow) directions in open (Left) versus minimally invasive (Right) techniques. The skin incision and lateral abdominal wall dissection (dashed arrow) are decreased in the latter approach

quadrant of L4, and it only rarely crosses the L4 vertebral body from posterior to anterior [9, 11]. Conceptually, the minimally invasive technique allows for both psoas dissection and cage insertion through the same pathway, thus requiring a shorter skin incision and less muscle disruption (Fig. 13.3, right). If spinal canal decompression is necessary, the transpsoas approach permits a relatively easy access, due to the small amount of posterior psoas fibers (that also contain the femoral nerve) located behind the posterior retractor blade. Moreover, this approach offers the major advantage of direct visualization of both the posteriorly displaced fragments and the dura mater to be decompressed [5].

Another advantage of the lateral transpsoas approach is the usage of a cage with wide footplate that can span the entire vertebral body and rest on the outer cortical ring, thus minimizing the risk of subsidence [10]. This, in turn, allows for a safer expansion of the cage, with better correction of the coronal and/or sagittal deformity [12].

The feasibility of this technique, particularly at L4, is determined by the position of the femoral nerve in the psoas muscle. Fortunately, the understanding of local anatomy and preoperative planning have improved with the increasing popularity of the lateral approach for degenerative pathology [11, 13–19]. If the femoral nerve is identified in the posterior quadrant at the L4–5 disc level [19] on the axial T2-weighted MRI images and the iliac crest height does not extend above the mid-vertebral body of L4 on lateral x-rays, the L4 minimally invasive corpectomy can be safely accomplished.

We prefer to perform the corpectomy first (including cage insertion), followed (or not) by decompression of the spinal canal. The first advantage is adequate cage placement. At the time of insertion, the cage will follow the path of least resistance: if the decompression is done first, the cage will tend to end up in a suboptimal posterior position, where the discectomy has been performed. The second advantage is that, if the PLL maintains some integrity, the posteriorly displaced fragments may be pulled anteriorly at the time of cage expansion, thus facilitating later removal. Finally, the cranial and caudal adjacent endplates are clearly defined by the cage footplates, thus minimizing the need for fluoroscopy to validate the extent of cranio-caudal decompression. The only potential disadvantage of pushing fracture fragments further in the canal can be avoided by removing enough bone during the corpectomy for the cage to insert easily.

The left side is typically used for most lateral approaches. We chose a right-sided approach in Patient 1 because the psoas muscle was relaxed (secondary to the coronal deformity) and the cage expansion would yield a better coronal correction.

The current surgical technique involves two discectomies by individual exposures, followed by corpectomy, with or without canal decompression. The challenge of the transpsoas dissection consists in opening the retractor from the inferior to the superior discectomy exposures in the direction of the psoas fibers. A potentially better retractor might involve two individual parts, one with three blades to expose the psoas and protect the retroperitoneum, and another to maintain the transpsoas exposure at and in-between the two discectomy sites.

Conclusion

The minimally invasive lateral transpsoas approach for lumbar corpectomy may offer a safe and less morbid alternative in patients with favorable anatomy.

References

1. Chou D, Lu DC. Mini-open transpedicular corpectomies with expandable cage reconstruction. Technical note. J Neurosurg Spine. 2011;14:71–7. https://doi.org/10.3171/2010.10.spine091009.
2. Lu DC, Lau D, Lee JG, Chou D. The transpedicular approach compared with the anterior approach: an analysis of 80 thoracolumbar corpectomies. J Neurosurgery Spine. 2010;12:583–91. https://doi.org/10.3171/2010.1.spine09292.
3. Smith ZA, Li Z, Chen NF, Raphael D, Khoo LT. Minimally invasive lateral extracavitary corpectomy: cadaveric evaluation model and report of 3 clinical cases. J Neurosurgery Spine. 2012;16:463–70. https://doi.org/10.3171/2012.2.SPINE11128.
4. Baaj AA, et al. Complications of the mini-open anterolateral approach to the thoracolumbar spine. J Clini Neurosci. 2012;19:1265–7. https://doi.org/10.1016/j.jocn.2012.01.026.
5. Uribe JS, Dakwar E, Cardona RF, Vale FL. Minimally invasive lateral retropleural thoracolumbar approach: cadaveric feasibility study and report of 4 clinical cases. Neurosurgery. 2011;68:32–9; discussion 39. https://doi.org/10.1227/NEU.0b013e318207b6cb.

6. Rihn JA, et al. A review of the TLICS system: a novel, user-friendly thoracolumbar trauma classification system. Acta Orthop. 2008;79:461–6. https://doi.org/10.1080/17453670710015436.
7. Vaccaro AR, et al. The thoracolumbar injury severity score: a proposed treatment algorithm. J Spinal Disord Tech. 2005;18:209–15.
8. Ozgur BM, Aryan HE, Pimenta L, Taylor WR. Extreme lateral interbody fusion (XLIF): a novel surgical technique for anterior lumbar interbody fusion. Spine J. 2006;6:435–43. https://doi.org/10.1016/j.spinee.2005.08.012.
9. Tender GC, Serban D. Genitofemoral nerve protection during the lateral retroperitoneal transpsoas approach. Neurosurgery. 2013;73:192–6; discussion 196-197. https://doi.org/10.1227/01.neu.0000431473.49042.95.
10. Pekmezci M, et al. Can a novel rectangular footplate provide higher resistance to subsidence than circular footplates? An ex vivo biomechanical study. Spine. 2012;37:E1177–81. https://doi.org/10.1097/BRS.0b013e3182647c0b.
11. Guerin P, et al. The lumbosacral plexus: anatomic considerations for minimally invasive retroperitoneal transpsoas approach. Surg Radiol Anat. 2012;34:151–7. https://doi.org/10.1007/s00276-011-0881-z.
12. Pekmezci M, et al. Comparison of expandable and fixed interbody cages in a human cadaver corpectomy model, part I: endplate force characteristics. J Neurosurg Spine. 2012;17:321–6. https://doi.org/10.3171/2012.7.spine12171.
13. Ahmadian A, Deukmedjian AR, Abel N, Dakwar E, Uribe JS. Analysis of lumbar plexopathies and nerve injury after lateral retroperitoneal transpsoas approach: diagnostic standardization. J Neurosurg Spine. 2012. https://doi.org/10.3171/2012.11.SPINE12755.
14. Banagan K, Gelb D, Poelstra K, Ludwig S. Anatomic mapping of lumbar nerve roots during a direct lateral transpsoas approach to the spine: a cadaveric study. Spine. 2011;36:E687–91. https://doi.org/10.1097/BRS.0b013e3181ec5911.
15. Benglis DM, Vanni S, Levi AD. An anatomical study of the lumbosacral plexus as related to the minimally invasive transpsoas approach to the lumbar spine. J Neurosurg Spine. 2009;10:139–44. https://doi.org/10.3171/2008.10.SPI08479.
16. Dakwar E, Ahmadian A, Uribe JS. The anatomical relationship of the diaphragm to the thoracolumbar junction during the minimally invasive lateral extracoelomic (retropleural/retroperitoneal) approach. J Neurosurg Spine. 2012;16:359–64. https://doi.org/10.3171/2011.12.SPINE11626.
17. Kepler CK, Bogner EA, Herzog RJ, Huang RC. Anatomy of the psoas muscle and lumbar plexus with respect to the surgical approach for lateral transpsoas interbody fusion. Eur Spine J. 2011;20:550–6. https://doi.org/10.1007/s00586-010-1593-5.
18. Lu S, et al. Clinical anatomy and 3D virtual reconstruction of the lumbar plexus with respect to lumbar surgery. BMC Musculoskelet Disord. 2011;12:76. https://doi.org/10.1186/1471-2474-12-76.
19. Uribe JS, Arredondo N, Dakwar E, Vale FL. Defining the safe working zones using the minimally invasive lateral retroperitoneal transpsoas approach: an anatomical study. J Neurosurg Spine. 2010;13:260–6. https://doi.org/10.3171/2010.3.SPINE09766.

Chapter 14
Thoracic Lateral Retropleural Discectomy

Gabriel Tender, Daniel Serban, Mihaela Florea, Adriana Constantinescu, and Kara Parikh

Introduction

Thoracic disc herniations can be very difficult to treat, particularly when calcified. Since the dural sac cannot be retracted, posterior access to central disc herniations is difficult or impossible without inflicting neurological deficits. The lateral approach offers the advantage of direct access to the disc herniations, whether central or paracentral, as well as their interface with the dura mater. A minimally invasive approach offers the same exposure and access, while minimizing morbidity. The minimally invasive lateral transthoracic retropleural approach can be performed throughout the thoracic spine below T5.

Electronic Supplementary Material The online version of this chapter https://doi.org/10.1007/978-3-319-71943-6_14. contains supplementary material, which is available to authorized users.

G. Tender (✉)
Louisiana State University, New Orleans, LA, USA

D. Serban • M. Florea
Department of Neurosurgery, "Bagdasar-Arseni" Hospital, Bucharest, Romania
e-mail: Dn.serban@gmail.com; florea.simona_mihaela@yahoo.com

A. Constantinescu
Universitatea de Medicina si Farmacie, Craiova, Romania
e-mail: Adriana_cnst@yahoo.com

K. Parikh
Department of Neurosurgery, Louisiana State University Health Sciences Center, New Orleans, LA, USA
e-mail: kparik@lsuhsc.edu

G. Tender (ed.), *Minimally Invasive Spine Surgery Techniques*,
https://doi.org/10.1007/978-3-319-71943-6_14

Indications

Patients present with signs of myelopathy and/or radiculopathy, concordant with the level of disc herniation identified on the MRI. Acute onset of symptoms may signal a soft, acute disc herniation, whereas chronic symptoms can occur with either soft or calcified herniations.

Contraindications

The T1–T5 vertebral bodies may be difficult to access via this approach, depending on the individual anatomy. We have successfully resected a T2–3 anterior meningioma, without performing a fusion, using this approach, but it was technically very demanding.

The position of the aorta, particularly if calcified, may mandate a right-sided approach.

Thoracic scarring from radiation or previous surgery represents a relative contraindication.

Preoperative Planning

Preoperative imaging, in the order performed, includes:

1. MRI: shows the disc herniation morphology and the amount of cord compression.
2. CT: shows the morphology of the disc herniation and the amount of calcification.
3. Lateral X-rays: show the loss of disc height and help identify the anatomy intraoperatively.

Surgical Technique

Patient Positioning

Regular intubation, without lung deflation, is performed. The patient is placed in lateral decubitus (preferably right, but it depends on the location of the disc herniation) and taped to the operating table in a fashion similar to the lateral transpsoas technique, previously described in the literature, with one obvious difference: the taping around the thorax avoids the site of the future skin incision. Patients' true lateral position is verified by AP fluoroscopy. In the patient presented in the

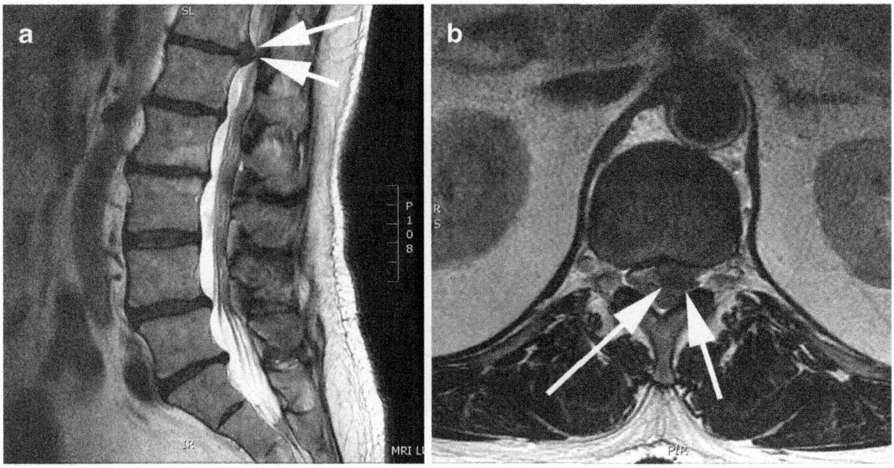

Fig. 14.1 Preoperative T2-weighted MRI, (**a**) sagittal and (**b**) axial images, showing a left T12-L1 paracentral disc herniation

Operative Video, the disc herniation was paracentral to the left, and therefore a left-sided approach was used (Fig. 14.1).

Exposure

The targeted disc is marked on the skin, based on the lateral fluoroscopic image, and a 6–7 cm skin incision is centered on the targeted segment, over the corresponding intercostal space. The cranial edge of the caudal rib is used to start detaching the parietal pleura from the anterior aspect of the rib. Most intercostal spaces allow for this dissection to be done with the index finger. The parietal pleura continues to be detached by following the rib posteriorly to its insertion. Once the vertebral body is palpated with the tip of the finger, the dilators and tubular retractors can be inserted to maintain exposure. If the intercostal space is too small to accommodate a finger or a retractor, part of the rib can be resected, but we have not had to this in over 30 cases performed to date.

We try to protect the parietal pleura integrity as much as possible, as it serves as a barrier between the retractor blades and the lung; however, in the depth, the parietal pleura is often adherent to the vertebral body and, upon placement of the retractor, the intrapleural space is usually exposed, with the edge of the lung often seen coming in and out of the field with each breath (as we mentioned, there is no need for dual-lumen intubation and lung deflation). Under lateral fluoroscopic guidance, the retractor is placed over the posterior aspect of the targeted disc, with the middle blade oriented posteriorly and the cranial and caudal blades opened towards the midbody of the adjacent vertebral bodies (Fig. 14.2). This placement facilitates easier orientation during surgery, obviating the need for repeated fluoroscopy. The

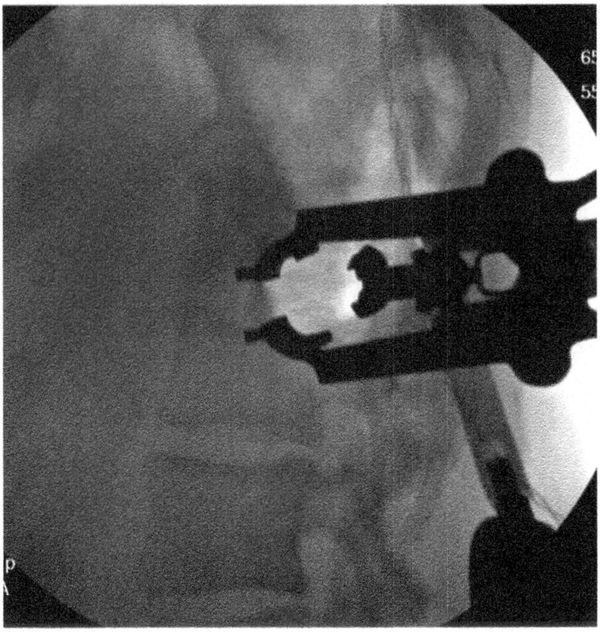

Fig. 14.2 Intraoperative lateral fluoroscopic image showing the retractor placement over the posterior aspect of the T12–L1 disc

fan-like retractor uses the parietal pleura as a protection layer and only the tip of the retractor comes in contact with, and keeps out of the operative field, the edge of the lung. Once the retractor is locked in place, the microscope is brought into the operative field.

Discectomy

The parietal pleura is coagulated over the disc of interest and then sharply transected with a long bayoneted knife. Once we confirm that the segmental vessels are not in the field, the disc is further exposed with the Bovie cautery. In order to access the disc, the head of the rib must be drilled off (exception: T12–L1, where the rib inserts on the body of T12 rather than the disc level). Once the disc is identified, the high-speed drill is used to remove the posterior caudal corner of the cranial vertebral body and the posterior cranial corner of the caudal vertebral body. The extent of this bony removal depends on the size and location of the disc herniation; in most cases, the resection does not need to extend past a third of the height of the vertebral body. The intervening posterior part of the disc is also removed with pituitary rongeurs. This creates a space in which the herniation will be pushed into.

Indeed, using the Penfield 4 and a long curette with a small cup (when more force is needed), the disc herniation is pushed anteriorly in the space created. It is important to custom order this instrument (the long, bayoneted, small-cup, straight

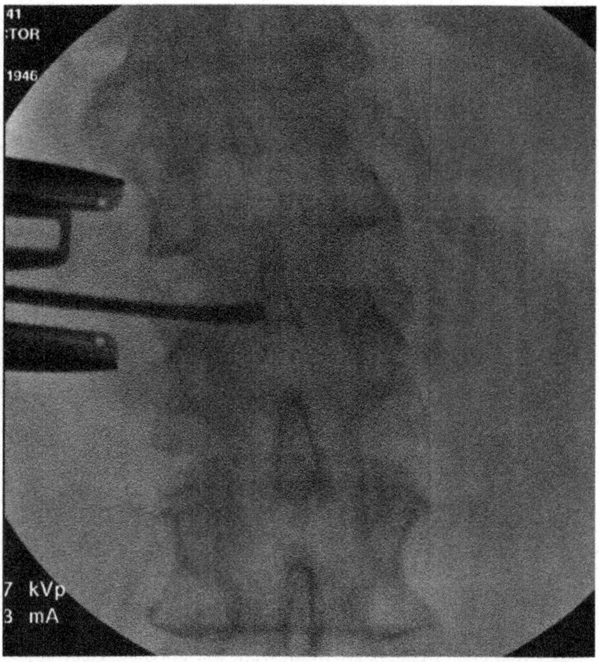

Fig. 14.3 Intraoperative AP fluoroscopic image showing the disc removal, as marked with a Penfield 4, extending to midline

curette) since it does not come in any of the regular sets. The posterior longitudinal ligament is a good anatomic landmark to understand where the dural sac is and where to look for the herniation.

We always confirm with an AP image that the decompression has gone deep enough, typically at or past the midline (Fig. 14.3). If not, further drilling in the depth is performed, to look for more herniated disc fragments. After a successful discectomy, the spinal sac can typically be seen re-expanding in its normal anatomical location. Postoperative MRI demonstrates the extent of the decompression (Fig. 14.4) and the CT shows the extent of bony removal (Fig. 14.5).

Closure

Before removing the retractor, we leave a regular Jackson-Pratt 7 flat drain in place, entering the chest posterior to the skin incision and with the tip against the lateral aspect of the cage. The drain not only evacuates any postoperative bleeding, but also can prevent a tension pneumothorax, if the lung parenchyma was violated and not recognized during surgery. Of course, if the lung injury was recognized during surgery, a formal chest tube should be inserted.

The wound is closed in anatomical layers, with interrupted 3-0 Vicryl for the hypodermis and 4-0 running Monocryl for the subcuticular layer.

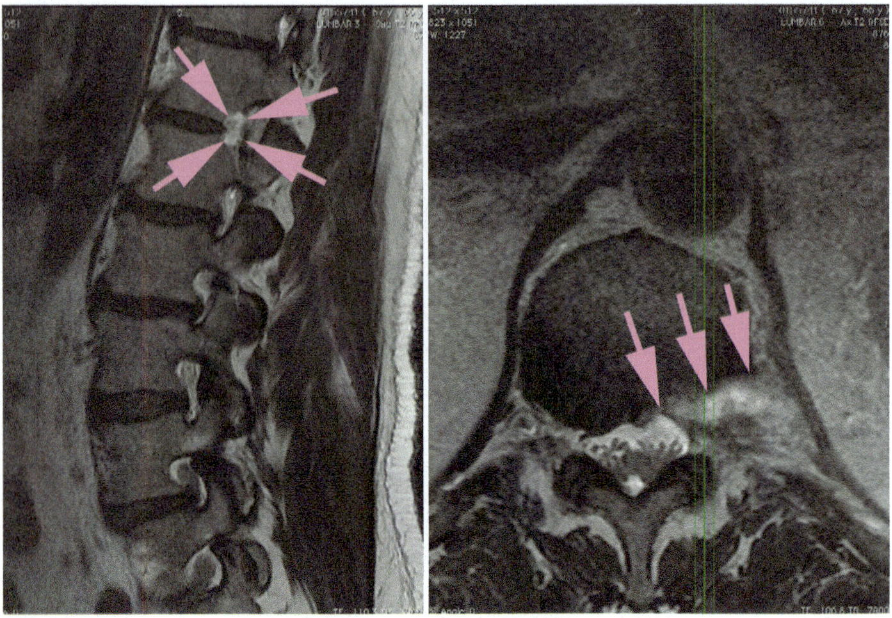

Fig. 14.4 Postoperative MRI showing the good surgical decompression, on (**a**) sagittal and (**b**) axial images

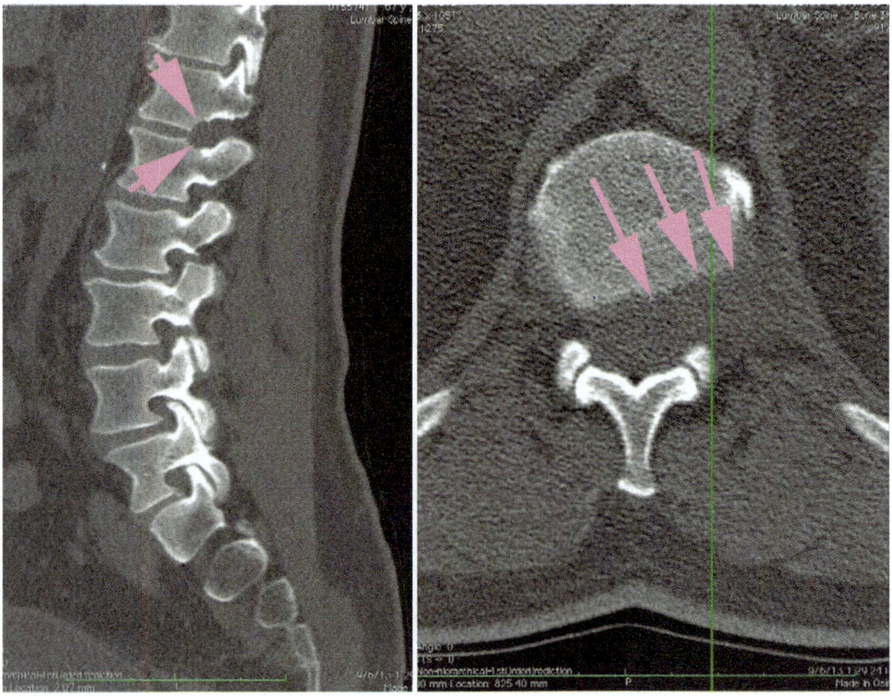

Fig. 14.5 Postoperative CT showing the extent of bony removal, on (**a**) sagittal and (**b**) axial images

Pearls and Pitfalls

High Thoracic Levels (T5–T6)

The main difference in these cases is the high position of the skin incision, in the axilla. In order to better expose this area, we recommend placing the ipsilateral arm on a sterile Mayo stand, so that the arm can be easily and independently mobilized out of the way during surgery. At these high levels, part of the medial aspect of the latissimus dorsi muscle may need to be either retracted or transected (and later re-approximated) and the long thoracic nerve must be protected, if identified.

Calcified Discs

These are probably among the most difficult cases for a spine surgeon (Fig. 14.6). The "calcified discs" are often osteophytes or segmental OPLL (ossified posterior longitudinal ligament) and the dura mater is absent at the level of the herniation. Therefore, a more extensive partial posterior corpectomy must be done, until normal vertebral body—dura mater interface is encountered. It is important to extend the bony removal not only in the cranio-caudal direction, but also in the depth, towards the contralateral side, until the osteophyte is completely detached from the vertebral body. The operative principle remains the same—a large enough cavity must be created anteriorly to allow for the osteophyte to be pushed into with the curette. It is common, in these cases, to have multiple areas of CSF extravasation, and occasionally nerve roots protrude in the operative field. We recommend advising the patients preoperatively of these risks and consent them for a lumbar drain at the time of discectomy, in case it is needed.

It is important to understand that, even though this can be an extremely difficult and frustrating approach, it offers the best chances of decompressing the spinal cord and nerves without (or with minimal) neurological deficits, since the posterior approaches face the same challenges (lack of dura mater, cord compression), but lack the necessary angle to access the osteophyte without dural retraction.

Complications

Neurological Injury/Dural Tears

The spinal cord and nerves are at risk during the separation of the disc herniation from the dura mater (or spinal cord, in case of segmental OPLL cases, in which there is no dura). In these cases, once the decompression is complete, a dural substitute is placed over the exposed spinal cord or nerves and a lumbar drain is inserted for 5–7 days. Dural sealants can be judiciously used in selected cases, with care not to compromise the spinal canal.

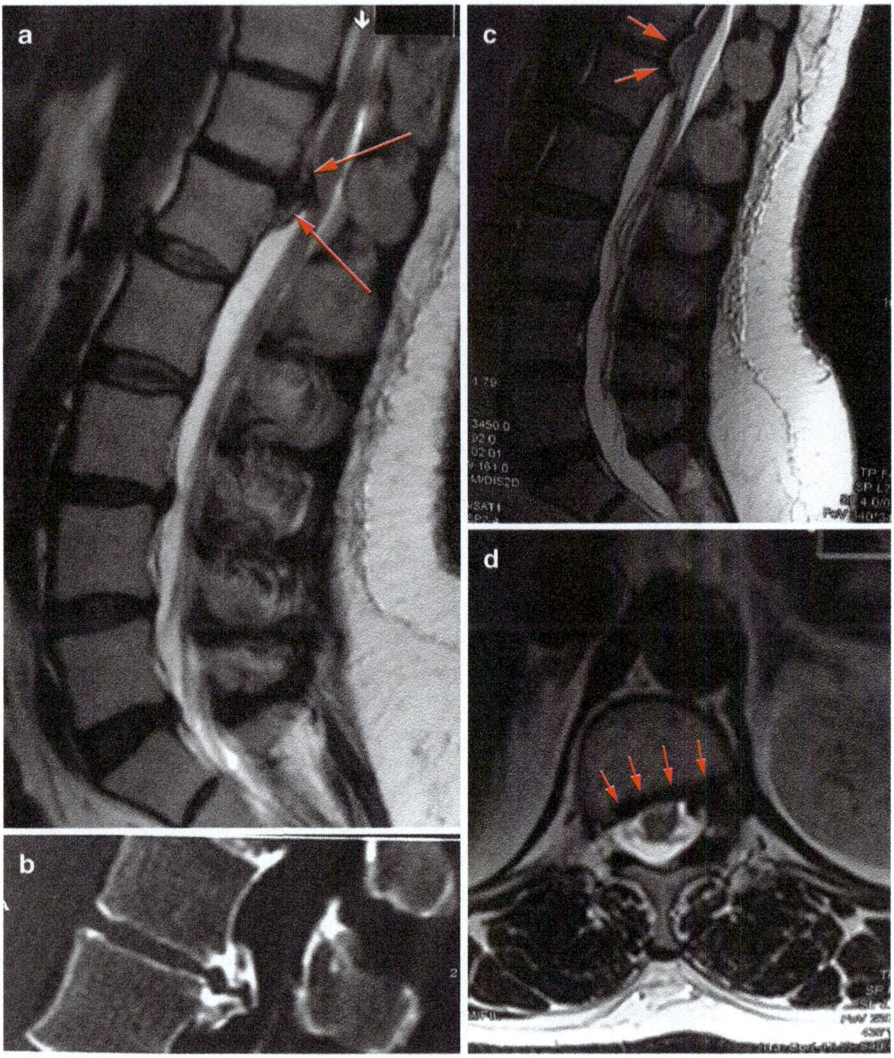

Fig. 14.6 A large T12–L1 osteophyte treated by a lateral minimally invasive approach. Preoperative (**a**) MRI and (**b**) CT, sagittal images, showing a large central osteophyte impinging on the spinal cord and creating severe spinal stenosis. Postoperative MRI, (**c**) sagittal and (**d**) axial images, showing the extent of bony removal and the successful surgical decompression

Lung Injury and Tension Pneumothorax

The lung can be inadvertently injured during the procedure with either the retractor or the high-speed drill. If suspected, filling the operative field with water and noticing air bubbles coming out during a Valsalva maneuver can easily detect this injury. If unrecognized intraoperatively, special attention during the postoperative care will discover that, after extubation, the bulb of the JP drain continues to fill with air very quickly. In this case, thoracic surgery should be consulted and a chest tube should be inserted. Unnoticed, the air leak from the lung injury can lead to tension pneumothorax and death.

Literature Review

The lateral approach offers certain advantages compared to the posterior approaches, such as less paraspinous muscle trauma and better access angle for the spinal canal decompression, particularly with centrally located disc herniations.

The minimally invasive retropleural approach for the thoracic and upper lumbar spine has been recently described [1–8] and the literature pertaining to this topic is relatively scarce.

Deviren et al. [8] described in 2011 their promising results in 12 consecutive patients who underwent a thoracic discectomy followed by an instrumented fusion.

Arts and Bartels [4] in 2014 compared the different approaches for thoracic disc herniations and concluded that medially located large calcified discs are best approached via an anterolateral approach, similar to our experience.

Yen and Uribe [1] in 2017 presented the largest patient series to date, 23 patients. The clinical results were good, but the surgeons were unable to remove 2 of the discs.

Conclusion

The minimally invasive lateral transthoracic retropleural approach may offer a safer and less morbid alternative in patients with disc herniations, particularly central or paracentral.

References

1. Yen CP, Uribe JS. Mini-open lateral retropleural approach for symptomatic thoracic disk herniations. Clin Spine Surg. 2017. https://doi.org/10.1097/bsd.0000000000000580.
2. Snyder LA, Smith ZA, Dahdaleh NS, Fessler RG. Minimally invasive treatment of thoracic disc herniations. Neurosurg Clin N Am. 2014;25:271–7. https://doi.org/10.1016/j.nec.2013.12.006.
3. Berjano P, et al. Transthoracic lateral retropleural minimally invasive microdiscectomy for T9-T10 disc herniation. Eur Spine J. 2014;23:1376–8. https://doi.org/10.1007/s00586-014-3369-9.
4. Arts MP, Bartels RH. Anterior or posterior approach of thoracic disc herniation? A comparative cohort of mini-transthoracic versus transpedicular discectomies. Spine J. 2014;14:1654–62. https://doi.org/10.1016/j.spinee.2013.09.053.

5. Falavigna A, Piccoli Conzatti L. Minimally invasive approaches for thoracic decompression from discectomy to corpectomy. J Neurosurg Sci. 2013;57:175–92.
6. Uribe JS, et al. Minimally invasive lateral approach for symptomatic thoracic disc herniation: initial multicenter clinical experience. J Neurosurg Spine. 2012;16:264–79. https://doi.org/10.3171/2011.10.spine11291.
7. Kasliwal MK, Deutsch H. Minimally invasive retropleural approach for central thoracic disc herniation. Minim Invasive Neurosurg. 2011;54:167–71. https://doi.org/10.1055/s-0031-1284400.
8. Deviren V, Kuelling FA, Poulter G, Pekmezci M. Minimal invasive anterolateral transthoracic transpleural approach: a novel technique for thoracic disc herniation. A review of the literature, description of a new surgical technique and experience with first 12 consecutive patients. J Spinal Disord Tech. 2011;24:E40–8. https://doi.org/10.1097/BSD.0b013e318220af6f.

Chapter 15
Percutaneous Thoracic Pedicle Screws

Parastou Fatemi, Anand Veeravagu, and John K. Ratliff

Introduction

Percutaneous thoracic pedicle screw insertion and fusion in the thoracic spine is a challenging minimally invasive procedure and necessitates pre-operative computer tomography (CT)- based planning and/or intra-operative fluoroscopic or CT navigation. Specific advantages of the percutaneous over open approach make it more appealing for select patients and experienced surgeons. Benefits of percutaneous thoracic instrumentation include reduced blood loss, decreased rate of infection, reduced length of hospital stay, earlier mobilization and return to work [1]. Improvement in intra-operative imaging techniques and robotics have increased the safety and accuracy of instrumentation placement. In this chapter we discuss the three options for instrumentation placement: x-ray fluoroscopy, navigated computer assisted, and robotic assisted.

Indications

The indications for percutaneous thoracic pedicle screw insertion and/or fusion are similar to those for open surgery with a few exceptions. Additionally, it should be noted that the surgeon should be prepared to convert to an open procedure should the need arise.

Trauma: Early surgical treatment of spinal injury following trauma is important in preserving neurologic function and even reversing loss of function. The current standard of treatment is open reduction and fixation of the spine; however, the percutaneous approach should be considered as a reasonable alternative especially in cases where the surgical team is trained in the technique, blood loss needs to be minimized,

P. Fatemi • A. Veeravagu • J.K. Ratliff (✉)
Department of Neurosurgery, Stanford University, Stanford, CA, USA
e-mail: parastou@stanford.edu; Anandv2@stanford.edu; jratliff@stanford.edu

G. Tender (ed.), *Minimally Invasive Spine Surgery Techniques*,
https://doi.org/10.1007/978-3-319-71943-6_15

and infection is a concern. Theodore et al. described using the percutaneous approach with c-arm fluoroscopy for five patients with unstable acute traumatic fractures and one osteoporotic burst fracture. Overall, 19 segments were fixated with 37 pedicle screws. Misplacement was grade II in 16% and grade III in 3%; none with neurologic consequence and none requiring revision or conversion to open procedure [2].

Osteomyelitis: In the thoracic spine, osteomyelitis may cause vertebral body collapse which may lead to excessive kyphosis and/or spinal cord compression. The percutaneous approach can be used to fixate the spine. If corpectomy is required, a combined open and percutaneous approach may be pursued, or an open surgical debridement may be required.

Neoplasm: The thoracic spine is the most common site of metastasis within the spinal column. Metastatic lesions can cause cord compression or result in significant kyphosis. The current guidelines recommend decompression and stabilization prior to radiation. Considering that patients with metastatic cancer often have limited life expectancy, minimally invasive surgery may be a better, less surgically morbid, option.

Depending on the surgical indication, diagnostic imaging may require x-rays, magnetic resonance imaging (MRI), and CT. For the purposes of surgery, preoperative CT and plain x-ray are essential. CT is imperative for assessing bone quality, determining extent of bony destruction (in cases of infection and neoplasm), and pedicle size. Standing X-rays aid in characterizing the degree of thoracic kyphosis and planning for sagittal correction, serving as a baseline image to be compared to post op follow up x-rays, and selecting distal and proximal endpoints of construct.

Contraindications

Contraindications for percutaneous thoracic pedicle screw insertion include general and specific issues. Generally, patients with many medical co-morbidities with high risk of peri-operative life-threatening complications, those with less than 3 months life expectancy, and poor bone quality/severe osteoporosis may not be considered surgical candidates. Additional contraindications include the need for surgical debridement of infection, resection of tumor mass, or decompression of the thoracic spinal cord.

Surgical Technique

Fluoroscopic Based Percutaneous Instrumentation [1]

Patient Positioning

The patient is first intubated under general anesthesia and appropriate access lines are established. The patient is positioned prone on a radiolucent prone lordotic table. Depending on the thoracic level of concern, arms are either placed out and bent at the elbow toward the head or tucked to the side. Care should be taken to sufficiently pad all pressure points. Motor and somatosensory potentials are established.

X-ray

Bi-planar or uni-planar fluoroscopy may be utilized for anatomic landmarks and appropriately positioned around the patient. Standard skin preparation and draping is then completed. Lateral fluoroscopy can be utilized to identify the level of interest. If this level is not clearly visible on lateral x-ray, then the surgeon may count from the sacrum to identify the level of interest. This level is marked on the skin.

A true anterior-posterior (AP) image is essential: the spinous process must be midline between the pedicles and the superior end plate is a single line (confirming the anterior and posterior portions of the end plate are in line).

A Jamshidi needle is used to identify the pedicle on AP fluoroscopy and the skin is marked. The incision is made lateral to the pedicle to allow for a lateral to medial trajectory through the skin and pedicle. The distance is typically 1 cm from the lateral wall of the pedicle, and the length of the incision is approximately 1 cm as well. However, patient's body habitus must be considered. The greater the depth of tissue, the more lateral the incision should be so that the Jamshidi needle can be successfully follow the angle of the pedicle. The incision is made through the skin and fascia.

Jamshidi Needle Placement

The Jamshidi needle is inserted through the skin incision and docked into the lateral aspect of the thoracic pedicle visualized on an AP X-ray (Fig. 15.1). Using a mallet, the needle is then directed to penetrate through the pedicle and into the vertebral

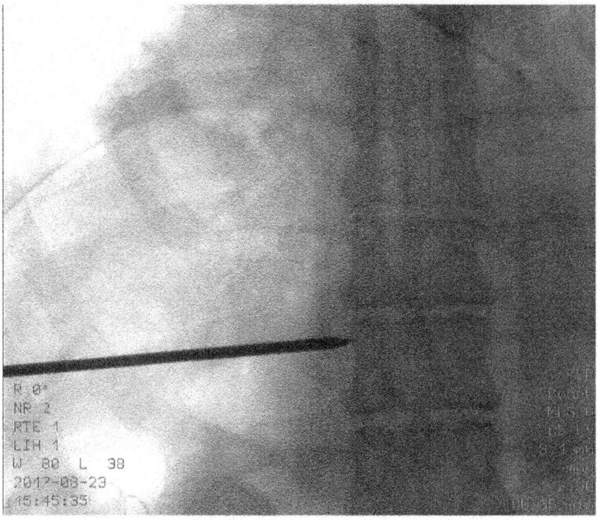

Fig. 15.1 AP fluoroscopic image showing the tip of the Jamshidi needle at the starting point, just lateral to the ring of the pedicle

body, to depth of approximately 20–25 mm. While the needle is being advanced, multiple x-rays are obtained in the lateral and AP views to ensure the needle remains on the correct trajectory and to avoid medial (and lateral) breach. This "AP only technique" requires understanding of the potential for medial breach during the advancement of the Jamshidi needle. The needle is in the correct position when the tip is in within the vertebral body on lateral x-ray and the needle has not breached the medial pedicle on AP x-ray. Correct placement should be confirmed with AP (Fig. 15.2) and lateral (Fig. 15.3) x-rays.

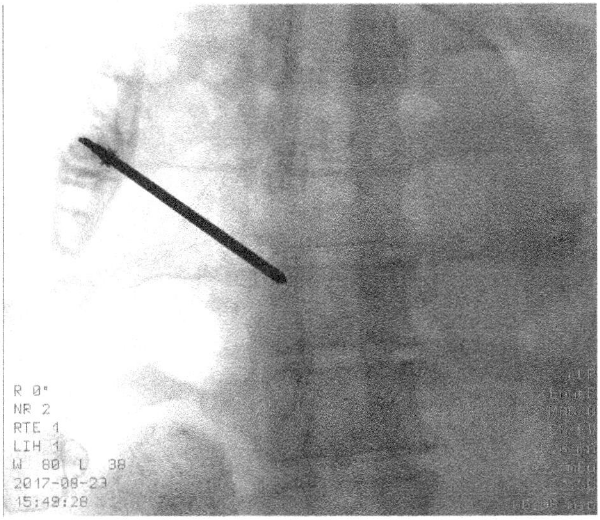

Fig. 15.2 AP fluoroscopic image showing the tip of the Jamshidi needle still within the pedicle ring, after advancing it for 2.5 cm from the starting point

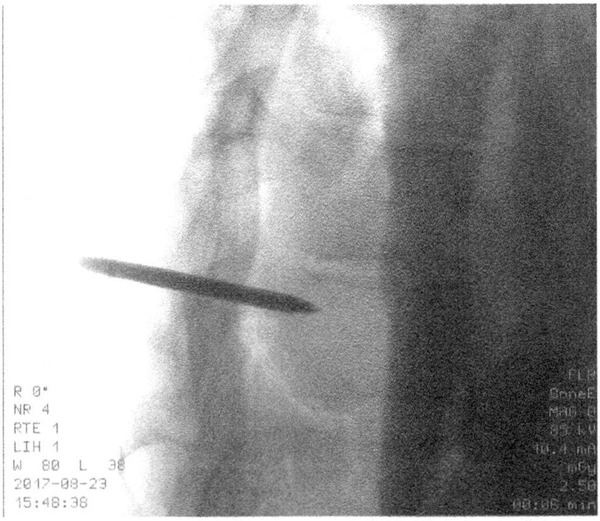

Fig. 15.3 Lateral fluoroscopic image showing the tip of the Jamshidi needle in the vertebral body

Guidewire Placement

The stylet is removed from the Jamshidi needle and Guidewire is inserted. The needle is then removed over the Guidewire. Another x-ray should be taken to confirm correct position of Guidewire. It is important to monitor and secure the Guidewire to prevent accidental advancement or pullout until the next step is performed.

Tap

Depending on the instrumentation system being used, dilators may be required prior to inserting a cannulated pedicle tap down the Guidewire trajectory. Again, serial x-rays are taken to ensure the guidewire remains in place and the tap is advanced along the correct trajectory within the pedicle. During advancement of the tap, bouncing of the guidewire will ensure the wire is not inadvertently advanced ventral. Lateral x-rays should be taken to ensure the ventral vertebral body has not been breached.

Pedicle Screw Placement

After tapping is complete, a previously selected pedicle screw of the appropriate size is inserted. The guidewire can be removed after the screw is at least midway through the pedicle. The screw is advanced until secure within the vertebral body, again ensuring it is in the correct position by serial x-rays. Guidewire management is critical in avoiding inadvertent ventral organ or vascular injury.

Rod Insertion

After all screws have been placed, rods may be inserted. The rod is inserted from the cranial to caudal direction, which is also the most to least superficial to the skin. Rod insertion may prove difficult depending on number of levels involved.

Compression or Distraction

After rods have been placed, the construct may be used to compress or distract the instrumented thoracic levels. X-ray is used to ensure adequate adjustment.

Final Tightening

Once a desired alignment and adjustment of space between levels is achieved, then the rods are tightened into the screws with appropriate caps. Final intra-operative x-ray is obtained.

Closure

The fascia and dermis are closed with interrupted Vicryl stitches. Running subcutaneous Monocryl is used for the skin closure. Surgical skin glue is applied to each incision.

Navigated, Computer Assisted

The advent of computer guidance and assistance has dramatically reduced the need for x-ray and fluoroscopy. In certain cases, such intra-operative 3-D X-ray or CT imaging systems may be of great utility in cannulating the pedicle. Almost all other portions of computer assisted MIS surgery remain the same when compared to fluoroscopy based instrumentation placement in that they are both guide wire dependent. The modification to the procedure detailed above in the case of computer assisted navigation is detailed below.

After patient position and standard preparation and draping is established—lateral x-ray may be used to identify the region of interest and the skin appropriately marked. A small 1 cm incision is made over the midline spinous process of the top most level of the surgical construct and a spinous process fixation clamp is attached. The 3-D x-ray is than brought into the operating room and a "spin" is completed to capture the region of interest. Once review of the scan indicates all regions of interest and pedicles are captured in the scan, the surgeon returns the operative field.

Using a navigation probe, verification of navigation accuracy is completed by confirming various known anatomical landmarks. Next, the navigation probe is used to identify the pedicle of interest in the navigation screen with an extension of the virtual tip to identify the transpedicular trajectory. The trajectory is saved and the skin is marked, and an incision is made similar to the procedure detailed prior.

At this point, a navigated drill guide is inserted through the incision and docked onto the facet, lining up with prior saved trajectory. A handheld drill set to 25 mm is inserted into the navigated drill guide and used to cannulate the pedicle. The drill guide is removed and a navigated tap is inserted. The navigated tap is removed and an appropriately sized screw is inserted.

The remainder of the procedure remains the same as described above in Sect. "Fluoroscopic Based Percutaneous Instrumentation [1]".

Robotic Assistance

The advent of robotic assistance has also dramatically changed options for percutaneous placement. There are of course multiple different types of robotic assistance available, however in this segment we discuss a general robotic system which results in cannulation of the pedicle and accurate Guidewire placement.

After patient position and standard preparation and draping is established—lateral x-ray may be used to identify the region of interest and the skin appropriately marked. A 1-cm incision is made over the mid-line spinous process of the top most level of the surgical construct and a spinous process fixation clamp is attached tightly. Then, the navigation is registered.

A small stab incision is made lateral to the spinous process on the skin along the pre-determined trajectory of the intended screw. Care must be taken to ensure the skin does not retract and impact the trajectory of instruments which will be used through the incision. Of note, the intended trajectory may be modified intra-operatively if needed.

The lateral incision is then lengthened enough to introduce the navigation system's cannula system without any retraction from the skin. Using a long scalpel, the incision is deepened through the fascia with the blade facing superiorly, scalpel is then removed and reinserted with the blade facing inferiorly.

When the appropriate opening is made, the cannula/dilator is inserted through the incision. Using a small amount of force and twisting/rotating technique, the dilator is advanced until bone is reached. Care should be taken not to place excessive pressure onto the dilator as this may cause skiving off the bone. The cannula is then stabilized on the bone and the inner dilator is removed and drill guide inserted and lightly tapped to engage the distal teeth into bone followed by harder tapping to secure it. If there is skin wrinkling at the drill guide/skin interface, then there may have been skiving of the bone and a new trajectory should be considered.

Next, the drill is inserted into the drill guide. The drill should be of proper length and depth measurement lines should be monitored while drilling. With drill bit about 1 cm off the bone, spin at maximum speed, then engage the bone and drill until appropriate depth is reached. Of note, the surgeon should not place much pressure as the drill primarily advances without much force. While drilling and removing the drill, care must be taken to ensure the trajectory remains similar to the pre-determined trajectory.

Next, a reduction tube is placed into the drill guide and advance into the drilled pilot hole. This may require some pressure and tactile should be noted until the bottom of the pilot hole is reached. Next, the guidance unit/arm is removed and a guidewire placed into the tube. At this time, the surgeon may tap and place a screw or proceed to prepare the next trajectory until all guidewires have been placed and then proceed with tapping and placing screws.

Pearls and Pitfalls

Ventral Vertebral Body Breach

This can be avoided three ways primarily. First, pre-operative selection of screw length. Second, upper thoracic regions T1–T4 have shorter vertebral body width; this should be considered in pre-operative planning of screw length. Third, intra-operative imaging helps ensure screws are placed appropriately through the pedicle and within the vertebral body without breach. Aggressive Guidewire management as described above can aid tremendously.

Small Pedicles

Upper thoracic vertebra have small pedicles, making it difficult for screw placement. The pedicle needs to be at least 3 mm, which can be assessed on pre-operative CT. In surgery, direct visualization of the pedicle in addition to changing angle of fluoroscopy to allow for bullseye view of the pedicle assist in successfully placing screw in a small pedicle.

If a small pedicle is attempted for needle and/or screw placement and the pedicle is burst, then the level has to be skipped. A supplemental laminar hook may be used to re-enforce the construct at this level.

In the event of pedicular size that prevents true cannulation, the "in-out-in" technique may be considered. In this modification, the Jamshidi needle is advanced through the transverse process and out into the costal transverse interval. The needle is then advanced into the lateral pedicle and down into the vertebral body, avoiding a medial breach secondary to a narrow proximal pedicle.

Changing Trajectory After Initial Needle Placement

If the trajectory following Jamshidi needle placement needs to be changed, the trajectory can be adjusted. The pedicle showed be tapped. Then, a smaller tap over the Guidewire can be used to change the angle of the trajectory, taking care not to excessively bend the Guidewire. Then the Guidewire should be removed and a new one placed on the correct path.

Passing Rod Over Multiple Levels

As the number of levels increases, placement of rod becomes more difficult. In our experience, placing the pre-bent rod from a cranial to caudal direction is best.

Medial Breach

If there is medial breach more than 4 mm, then there is concern for dural tear and possible neurologic injury. The procedure may need to be converted to open to repair the dural tear. Breaches less than 2 mm are well tolerated.

Complications

Anterior Breach of Screws

Due to vascular structures close to the thoracic vertebra, including the aorta on the left side, anterior breach may require revision. However, if breach is minimal and not adjacent to a vascular structure, no intervention is needed.

Neurologic Injury

This can occur with a medial breach, especially if greater than 4 mm, during any part of the procedure (needle placement, guidewire, tap, screw placement). Conversion to an open procedure may be required for dural repair.

Construct Failure With or Without Screw Pullout

Patients with osteoporosis have greater risk of screw pullout. Construct failure will often require revision surgery. Thought should be placed into the length of construct, screw size, and pre-operative osteoporosis treatment.

Deep Venous Thrombosis, Pulmonary Embolism

Immobilization during surgery and failure to mobilize patients early post op increases risk for DVTs and PEs. All patients should be on chemical DVT prophylaxis and mobile by post op day one. Prolonged anticoagulation will be needed with DVT/PE.

Urinary Tract Infection

Foley catheter is placed prior to surgery and should be removed as soon as post op day 1 when patient has mobilized to decrease catheter associated UTI.

Wound Infection

This risk increases in patients with uncontrolled blood glucose levels. Often infections are superficial and may be treated by antibiotics; however, deep infections require washout.

Literature Review

There is no prospective comparative study of open compared with percutaneous thoracic pedicle screw placement. Several studies have shown its efficacy in trauma/fracture, deformity, and neoplasm. Cadaveric studies have shown accuracy of screw placement with the percutaneous approach [3]. The advantages of the minimally invasive approach include lower blood loss, lower infection rates, reduced length of stay, earlier mobilization and return to work.

Li et al. wrote a great review of the procedure in their 2010 paper *Techniques, challenges and indications for percutaneous pedicle screw fixation* [1]. The percutaneous method has also been described in several textbooks, including AOSPINE Manual: Principles and Techniques [4], Handbook of Spine Surgery [5], Minimally Invasive Spine Surgery [6], and Neurosurgical Operative Atlas: Spine and Peripheral Nerves [7]. The method is also described by Oppenheimer and McDonnell in e-Neurosurgery.

Conclusions

Percutaneous thoracic pedicle screw insertion and fusion in thoracic spine may be challenging; however, the advantages of the procedure in terms of surgical morbidity over the open approach make it an advantageous option for select diagnoses and patients. A number of techniques exist to achieve percutaneous thoracic instrumentation placement, the latest being robotic, navigated and computer assisted.

References

1. Mobbs R, Sivabalan P, Li J. Technique, challenges and indications for percutaneous pedicle screw fixation. J Clin Neurosci. 2011;18(6):741–9.
2. Kakarla U, Little A, Chang S, Sonntag V, Theodore N. Placement of percutaneous thoracic pedicle screws using neuronavigation. World Neurosurg. 2010;74(6):606–10.
3. Hardin C, Nimjee S, Karikari I, Agarwal A, Fessler R, Isaacs R. Percutaneous pedicle screw placement in the thoracic spine: a cadaveric study. Asian J Neurosurg. 2013;8(3):153–6.
4. Langlotz F, Nolte L. AOSpine manual: principles and techniques, vol. 1. Davos: AO Publishing; 2007.
5. Baaj A, Mummanei P, Uribe J, Vaccaro A, Greenberg M. Chap. 60: Percutaneous pedicle screw placement. In: Handbook of spine surgery. New York: Thieme; 2016.
6. Hartl R, Korge A. Minimally invasive spine surgery - techniques, evidence, and controversies. Davos-Platz: AOSpine; 2012.
7. Wolfa C, Resnick D. Neurosurgical operative atlas: spine and peripheral nerves. New York: Thieme; 2017.

Chapter 16
Thoracic Lateral Retropleural Corpectomy

Gabriel Tender, Durga R. Sure, Yasser Badr, Clifford Crutcher, and Lindsay Lasseigne

Introduction

The standard surgical approach for thoracic corpectomy is usually performed by the thoracic surgeon and involves extensive thoracic wall dissection, rib removal, and unilateral lung deflation, thus resulting in significant morbidity. The minimally invasive surgery (MIS) option for the lateral transthoracic approach has been successfully used in the thoracic spine (T5–T12) with good results, since the dissection for exposing these levels is mostly extrapleural. We describe this minimally invasive lateral transthoracic extrapleural technique, in which the incision is about 2–3-in. long, one rib is partially resected, the dissection is mostly extrapleural, and the lung is not deflated. At our institution, the spine surgeon performs this approach, although a thoracic surgeon is available, if needed.

Electronic Supplementary Material The online version of this chapter https://doi.org/10.1007/978-3-319-71943-6_16. contains supplementary material, which is available to authorized users.

G. Tender (✉)
Louisiana State University, New Orleans, LA, USA

D.R. Sure
Essentia Health, Duluth, MN, USA

Y. Badr
Badr Brain and Spine, Los Angeles, CA, USA

C. Crutcher • L. Lasseigne
Department of Neurosurgery, Louisiana State University Health Sciences Center, New Orleans, LA, USA
e-mail: ccrutc@lsuhsc.edu; llasse@lsuhsc.edu

G. Tender (ed.), *Minimally Invasive Spine Surgery Techniques*,
https://doi.org/10.1007/978-3-319-71943-6_16

Indications

The minimally invasive lateral transthoracic retropleural approach can be performed for T5 through T12 corpectomy. The lesions affecting the vertebral body that needs to be resected can be traumatic, tumoral, or infectious.

Trauma

The classification and indications for surgical treatment in thoracolumbar fractures have evolved over the past 50 years along with the diagnostic capabilities. Currently, the thoracolumbar injury classification and severity (TLICS) system takes into account fracture morphology, posterior ligamentous complex (PLC) integrity, and neurological status [1, 2]. In patients with comminuted vertebral body fractures and posterior ligamentous complex disruption, a circumferential (anterior and posterior) fixation is recommended.

Tumors

Primary or metastatic tumors can affect the thoracic vertebral bodies and may result in either loss of vertebral body height with kyphotic deformity and/or anterior spinal cord compression. These tumors can be successfully approached via the minimally invasive lateral transthoracic retropleural approach. However, if the tumor extends into the pedicles and/or has a significant component in the lateral or posterior spinal canal, the postero-lateral approach may provide better circumferential decompression of the canal.

Infection

In cases of discitis, the minimally invasive lateral transthoracic retropleural approach offers an excellent route to perform an extensive disc debridement and possibly decompression of an anterior epidural abscess compressing the spinal sac. We prefer not to use instrumentation in these cases until the infection is controlled. However, occasionally, there is extensive destruction of the adjacent vertebral bodies and major neurological deficits due to compression of the spinal cord. Almost invariably, these patients also present with significant kyphotic deformity. In this situation, a 2-level corpectomy with decompression of the spinal canal and reconstruction with an expandable cage, followed by posterior instrumentation with or without osteotomies, may become mandatory.

Contraindications

The T1–T5 vertebral bodies may be difficult to access via this approach, depending on the individual anatomy. We have successfully resected a T2–3 anterior meningioma, without performing a fusion, using this approach, but it was technically very demanding.

The position of the aorta, particularly if calcified, may mandate a right-sided approach.

Thoracic scarring represents a relative contraindication.

Preoperative Planning

Preoperative imaging, in the order performed, includes:

1. Lateral and AP X-rays: show the loss of vertebral body height and the local sagittal and/or coronal deformity;
2. CT: shows the morphology of the fractures or the amount of bony destruction in infections or tumors.
3. MRI: shows the amount of cord compression and the status of the posterior ligamentous complex (on STIR images)

Angiography can be useful in assessing vascular tumors and embolization can be performed at that time. Although uncommon, it can also be used to determine the level of origin for the Adamkiewicz artery, in order to avoid that level during surgery.

Surgical Technique

Patient Positioning

Regular intubation, without lung deflation, is performed. The patient is placed in lateral decubitus (preferably right, but it depends on whether there is coronal deformity) and taped to the operating table in a fashion similar to the lateral transpsoas technique, previously described in the literature, with one obvious difference: the taping around the thorax avoids the site of the future skin incision. Patients' true lateral position is verified by AP fluoroscopy.

Exposure

The targeted vertebral body is marked on the skin, based on the lateral fluoroscopic image, and a 6–9 cm skin incision is centered on the targeted segment, over the corresponding rib (Video 16.1, Video 16.2). After local hemostasis, the rib is exposed and completely detached from the surrounding tissues, including the parietal pleura, not only under the skin incision, but also 2–3 cm in front and behind it (since the skin can easily be retracted over the rib in both directions). The rib is then transected with the rib cutter over the entire previously detached length. Resecting the rib more anteriorly under the skin incision facilitates a better angle to visualize and possibly decompress the spinal canal, whereas resecting the rib more posteriorly under the skin incision allows for the dissecting finger to reach the vertebral body during the next step.

The parietal pleura is detached by blunt finger dissection from the remainder of the resected rib, as well as the ribs above and below. Following the ribs proximally, the finger (or a Kittner dissector) eventually encounters the junction with the vertebral body. We try to protect the parietal pleura integrity as much as possible, as it serves as a barrier between the retractor blades and the lung; however, in the depth, the parietal pleura is often adherent to the vertebral body and, upon placement of the retractor, the intrapleural space is usually exposed, with the edge of the lung often seen coming in and out of the field with each breath (as we mentioned, there is no need for dual-lumen intubation and lung deflation). In trauma patients with pleural fluid, the moment of intrapleural space exposure may be associated with a gush of pleural fluid in the operative field, mimicking a vascular injury. The retractor is placed over the fractured vertebral body (on lateral fluoroscopy), with the cranial and caudal blades lined up with the direction of the vertebral body (and the future cage) and above and below the corresponding discs, the posterior blade lined up with the posterior wall of the vertebral body, and the anterior fan-like retractor lined up with the anterior vertebral body line. This placement facilitates easier orientation during surgery, obviating the need for repeated fluoroscopy. The fan-like retractor uses the parietal pleura as a protection layer and only the tip of the retractor comes in contact with, and keeps out of the operative field, the edge of the lung. Once the retractor is locked in place, the microscope is brought into the operative field. The segmental vessels at the level of interest are isolated and initially protected. Care must be exercised before transecting these vessels, particularly at the lower thoracic levels, in order to ensure that the Adamkiewicz artery does not originate from that segmental artery. We recommend temporary soft occlusion of the exposed segmental artery (e.g., with a Kittner), for about 10′; if no MEP changes are reported by neuromonitoring, than it should be safe to transect the vessel. It is important to use MEP, since SSEPs will not be changed in case of Adamkiewicz artery occlusion.

Corpectomy

At this time, the discs above and below the level of interest are marked with spinal needles inserted preferably at the junction between the anterior third and posterior two-thirds on the lateral fluoroscopic image. The discectomies are then centered on these marks, aiding with proper future positioning of the cage in the anterior part of the intervertebral space and in line with the vertebral bodies above and below. Depending on the size of the vertebral bodies, the discectomies may be designed to accommodate a 19 mm or 22 mm cage footplate. We prefer to perform a fairly extensive discectomy and endplate preparation (the endplates of the cranial and caudal vertebral bodies, of course, since the endplates of the diseased segment will be removed during the corpectomy), because at this stage there is very little bleeding. We also penetrate the contralateral annulus at both disc levels with a sharp Cobb; attention must be paid not to injure the aorta on the contralateral side during this maneuver. The width and length of the footplates are determined at this time with appropriate sizers.

After this, the actual corpectomy is performed. The corpectomy has to be wide enough to easily accommodate the core of the cage, so that no fragments get pushed posteriorly in the spinal canal. We typically leave a thin layer of bone in the contralateral aspect of the resected vertebral body, since that will not interfere with cage placement and at the same time will minimize morbidity from the contralateral tissues or vessels. The depth of the corpectomy can be easily checked on the AP fluoroscopy; in fact, we keep the fluoroscopic machine in place during this part of the procedure, and use the microscope from an angle to access the operative field.

The corpectomy also has to be done fast, since the cancellous bone (or tumoral bone) can bleed briskly at this time. For that reason, we use osteotomes to remove most of the bone, safely away from the spinal canal, and only use the high-speed drill for the second part of the osteotomy, when decompressing the spinal canal (if necessary), *after* cage insertion.

A thin, expandable trial is used at this time to measure the distance between the endplates and determine the desire height of the cage to be built. Once that is determined, we place Floseal over the exposed cancellous (or tumoral) bone to control the bleeding and we leave it in place while the endplates undergo the final preparation, the footplates are sized (if not already done) and the cage is built on the back table.

Cage Insertion

Once the cage is built, the Floseal is washed off and two sliding blades are placed in the previously created discectomies. The cage is filled with graft material and then inserted between the two sliding blades under AP fluoroscopic guidance. The cage is advanced until its' core is lined up with the spinous processes above and below. A lateral fluoroscopic image is taken to confirm the adequate placement, and the sliding blades are removed. The cage inserter is then used to start expanding the cage. We prefer to do the expansion under AP fluoroscopy; we take a shot before expansion and then every 4–5 turns of the handle, until the desired height is achieved. This is also signaled by the tactile feel of increasing difficulty to expand the cage. We prefer to test the cage by pulling on it; it should not move at all. The cage inserter is then detached from the cage and further graft material can be packed into the cage (since the original graft got loose during cage expansion).

Canal Decompression

This step is only necessary if there is canal compromise and spinal cord impingement by fracture fragments, tumor, or abscess. At this time, the retractor is slightly angled from anterior to posterior (20–30°) while holding downward pressure to maintain contact with the bone. The high-speed drill is used to thin out the fragments protruding in the spinal canal and a long, bayoneted, small-cup, straight curette is used to separate the posterior longitudinal ligament from the dura mater and push the ligament along with the remainder of the fractured fragments anteriorly, away from the spinal canal. It is important to custom order this instrument (the long, bayoneted, small-cup, straight curette) since it does not come in any of the regular sets. Copious bleeding from the epidural venous plexus usually occurs and can be controlled with gelatin thrombin hemostatic sealants and gentle pressure. The decompression is continued in the cranial and caudal direction until the respective discs are encountered, as well as towards the contralateral side, until the level of the contralateral pedicle is reached, on the AP fluoroscopic image. Once the decompression is completed, the dura mater of the spinal sac typically expands into the operative field, back into its' normal anatomic position.

Closure

Once the canal is decompressed, further graft material can be added anteriorly and laterally around the cage, but with great care not to come in contact with the dura mater and potentially compress the spinal cord.

Before removing the retractor, we leave a regular Jackson-Pratt 7 flat drain in place, entering the chest posterior to the skin incision and with the tip against the lateral aspect of the cage. The drain not only evacuates any postoperative bleeding, but also can prevent a tension pneumothorax, if the lung parenchyma was violated and not recognized during surgery. Of course, if the lung injury was recognized during surgery, a formal chest tube should be inserted.

We also try to provide a watertight closure of the intercostal muscles as an individual layer. The resected rib can be reattached in its original position with titanium plates, but we have not done that, since the associated morbidity is minimal. The rest of the wound is closed in anatomical layers, with interrupted 3-0 Vycril for the hypodermis and 4-0 running Monocryl for the subcuticular layer.

Pearls and Pitfalls

High Thoracic Levels (T5–T6)

The main difference in these cases is the high position of the skin incision, in the axilla. In order to better expose this area, we recommend placing the ipsilateral flexed arm on a sterile Mayo stand coming from the cranial end of the table (where anesthesia normally is), so that the arm can be easily and independently mobilized out of the way during surgery. At these high levels, part of the medial aspect of the latissimus dorsi muscle may need to be either retracted or transected (and later re-approximated) and the long thoracic nerve must be protected, if identified.

Discectomy and Endplate Preparation

Since the discs have a bi-convex shape (unless severely degenerated, in which case they become flat), endplate preparation must be done respecting its' concave shape. The best preparation, in our opinion, is done with a wide Cobb (20 or 22 mm for the lower thoracic spine, 16 or 18 mm for the mid and upper thoracic spine) that follows the dissection plane between the disc and the endplate. As the Cobb follows the concave surface of the endplate, the direction of the shaft changes from cranially angled (initially) to straight (as the tip of the Cobb passes the midpoint of the disc). If this direction is not changed, there is a risk of endplate and vertebral body violation in the deep (contralateral) half of the vertebral body.

Corpectomy

The corpectomy has to be wide enough to easily accommodate the core of the cage, so that no fragments get pushed posteriorly in the spinal canal. We typically leave a thin layer of bone in the contralateral aspect of the resected vertebral body, since that will not interfere with cage placement and at the same time will minimize morbidity from the contralateral tissues and/or vessels.

The corpectomy also has to be done fast, since the cancellous bone (or tumoral bone) can bleed briskly at this time. For that reason, we use osteotomes to remove most of the bone, safely away from the spinal canal, and only use the high-speed drill for the second part of the osteotomy, when decompressing the spinal canal (if necessary), *after* cage insertion.

Bleeding from the cancellous (or tumoral) bone can be controlled with Floseal, which can be left in place while the endplates undergo the final preparation and the footplates are sized.

We prefer to perform the corpectomy first (including cage insertion), followed (or not) by decompression of the spinal canal. The first advantage is adequate cage placement At the time of insertion, the cage will follow the path of least resistance: if the decompression is done first, the cage will tend to end up in a suboptimal posterior position, where the discectomy has been performed. The second advantage is that, if the PLL maintains some integrity, the posteriorly displaced fragments may be pulled anteriorly at the time of cage expansion, thus facilitating later removal. Finally, the cranial and caudal adjacent endplates are clearly defined by the cage footplates, thus minimizing the need for fluoroscopy to validate the extent of cranio-caudal decompression. The only potential disadvantage of pushing fracture fragments further in the canal can be avoided by removing enough bone during the corpectomy for the cage to insert easily.

Complications

Neuro-Vascular Injury

The spinal cord is at risk during the insertion of the cage, if an insufficient corpectomy has been performed. However, if the decompression is performed before cage insertion, the cage almost invariably follows the path of least resistance and ends up too posteriorly located.

The aorta is rarely injured, either directly during the exposure, or on the contralateral side during penetration of the contralateral annulus.

Care must be exercised before transecting the segmental vessels, particularly at the lower thoracic levels, in order to ensure that the Adamkiewicz artery does not originate from that segmental artery. We recommend temporary soft occlusion of the exposed segmental artery (e.g., with a Kittner), for about 10′; if no MEP changes are reported by neuromonitoring, than it should be safe to transect the vessel. It is important to use MEP, since SSEPs will not be changed in case of Adamkiewicz artery occlusion.

Dural Tears

Occasionally, a sharp fracture fragment can penetrate the posterior longitudinal ligament and the dura and, upon removal, can lead to CSF extravasation. More commonly, the surgeon inadvertently injures the dura at the time of fracture fragment removal. In either case, the dural tear is usually not amenable to direct repair. Instead, we recommend gentle tamponade with Gelfoam followed by DuraSeal, and placement of a lumbar drain for 5–7 days.

Inadequate Placement of the Cage

This should be recognized intraoperatively. Typically, the cage is either placed to far posteriorly, especially if the canal decompression is performed before cage insertion, or is placed at an oblique angle against the endplates. Either way, when recognized on the lateral fluoroscopic image, the cage can be repositioned more anteriorly or at the correct angle, respectively.

Lung Injury and Tension Pneumothorax

The lung can be inadvertently injured during the procedure with either the retractor, the high-speed drill, the osteotomes, or any other instrument. If suspected, filling the operative field with water and noticing air bubbles coming out during a Valsalva maneuver can easily detect this injury. If unrecognized intraoperatively, special attention during the postoperative care will discover that, after extubation, the bulb of the JP drain continues to fill with air very quickly. In this case, thoracic surgery should be consulted and a chest tube should be inserted. Unnoticed, the air leak from the lung injury can lead to tension pneumothorax and death.

Literature Review

The lateral approach offers certain advantages compared to the posterior approaches, such as less paraspinous muscle trauma and better access angle for the spinal canal decompression, particularly with centrally located fragments. However, the preference of the approach is still heavily dependent on surgeons' experience [3, 4].

Initial studies showed the feasibility of the minimally invasive technique and the early results [5–10].

Follow-up studies showed good results with this technique [11–16], although no prospective studies have been performed.

Conclusion

The minimally invasive lateral transpsoas approach for lumbar corpectomy may offer a safe and less morbid alternative in patients with favorable anatomy.

References

1. Vaccaro AR, et al. Reliability of a novel classification system for thoracolumbar injuries: the thoracolumbar injury severity score. Spine (Phila Pa 1976). 2006;31:S62–9; discussion S104. https://doi.org/10.1097/01.brs.0000218072.25964.a9.
2. Vaccaro AR, et al. The thoracolumbar injury severity score: a proposed treatment algorithm. J Spinal Disord Tech. 2005;18:209–15.
3. Lu DC, Lau D, Lee JG, Chou D. The transpedicular approach compared with the anterior approach: an analysis of 80 thoracolumbar corpectomies. J Neurosurg Spine. 2010;12:583–91. https://doi.org/10.3171/2010.1.spine09292.
4. Archavlis E, Papadopoulos N, Ulrich P. Corpectomy in destructive thoracolumbar spine disease: cost-effectiveness of 3 different techniques and implications for cost reduction of delivered care. Spine (Phila Pa 1976). 2015;40:E433–8. https://doi.org/10.1097/brs.0000000000000782.
5. Baaj AA, et al. Complications of the mini-open anterolateral approach to the thoracolumbar spine. J Clin Neurosci. 2012;19:1265–7. https://doi.org/10.1016/j.jocn.2012.01.026.
6. Uribe JS, Dakwar E, Cardona RF, Vale FL. Minimally invasive lateral retropleural thoracolumbar approach: cadaveric feasibility study and report of 4 clinical cases. Neurosurgery. 2011;68:32–9; discussion 39. https://doi.org/10.1227/NEU.0b013e318207b6cb.
7. Uribe JS, et al. Minimally invasive surgery treatment for thoracic spine tumor removal: a mini-open, lateral approach. Spine (Phila Pa 1976). 2010;35:S347–54. https://doi.org/10.1097/BRS.0b013e3182022d0f.
8. Smith WD, et al. Minimally invasive surgery for traumatic spinal pathologies: a mini-open, lateral approach in the thoracic and lumbar spine. Spine. 2010;35:S338–46. https://doi.org/10.1097/BRS.0b013e3182023113.
9. Ogden AT, et al. Cadaveric evaluation of minimally invasive posterolateral thoracic corpectomy: a comparison of 3 approaches. J Spinal Disord Tech. 2009;22:524–9. https://doi.org/10.1097/BSD.0b013e31818e5488.
10. Kim DH, et al. Minimally invasive posterolateral thoracic corpectomy: cadaveric feasibility study and report of four clinical cases. Neurosurgery. 2009;64:746–52; discussion 752-753. https://doi.org/10.1227/01.neu.0000340783.83964.27.
11. Holland CM, Bass DI, Gary MF, Howard BM, Refai D. Thoracic lateral extracavitary corpectomy for anterior column reconstruction with expandable and static titanium cages: clinical outcomes and surgical considerations in a consecutive case series. Clin Neurol Neurosurg. 2015;129:37–43. https://doi.org/10.1016/j.clineuro.2014.11.022.
12. Park MS, Deukmedjian AR, Uribe JS. Minimally invasive anterolateral corpectomy for spinal tumors. Neurosurg Clin N Am. 2014;25:317–25. https://doi.org/10.1016/j.nec.2013.12.009.
13. Lau D, Song Y, Guan Z, La Marca F, Park P. Radiological outcomes of static vs expandable titanium cages after corpectomy: a retrospective cohort analysis of subsidence. Neurosurgery. 2013;72:529–39; discussion 528-529. https://doi.org/10.1227/NEU.0b013e318282a558.
14. Ahmadian A, Uribe JS. Mini-open lateral retro-pleural thoracic corpectomy for osteomyelitis. Neurosurg Focus. 2013;35:Video 17. https://doi.org/10.3171/2013.v2.focus13221.
15. Lall RR, Smith ZA, Wong AP, Miller D, Fessler RG. Minimally invasive thoracic corpectomy: surgical strategies for malignancy, trauma, and complex spinal pathologies. Minim Invasive Surg. 2012;2012:213791. https://doi.org/10.1155/2012/213791.
16. Khan SN, Cha T, Hoskins JA, Pelton M, Singh K. Minimally invasive thoracolumbar corpectomy and reconstruction. Orthopedics. 2012;35:e74–9. https://doi.org/10.3928/01477447-20111122-04.

Chapter 17
Posterior Cervical Foraminotomy

George M. Ghobrial and Allan D. Levi

Introduction

The posterior cervical foraminotomy (PCF) approach was first described by Spurling and Scoville for the treatment of posterolateral cervical soft disc herniations with concordant radiculopathy [1]. Subsequently, multiple surgical series have demonstrated a high rate of clinical success using this approach, citing a low complication rate, morbidity, rate of disk recurrence, and rate of reoperation [2–6]. The ideal management of cervical radiculopathy is still contested. Proponents of the ventral approach argue that the anterior discectomy and fusion (ACF) has less postoperative pain and cervical deformity due to the avoidance of posterior muscular dissection, providing a wider exposure of the pathology affording safe disc removal, as well as a lower rate of iatrogenic nerve injury [7, 8]. One important drawback of the ACF is that it does not preserve mobility. The cervical disc arthroplasty, an alternative anterior option is motion-sparing, but still carries risks inherent to an anterolateral approach. One of the most common complications is dysphagia which can persist after surgery while the least common and most concerning of outcomes is injury to the esophagus or vertebral artery [9]. In the postoperative months, the risks of graft subsidence and pseudoarthrosis are unique to the anterior approach [7]. Moreover, after successful fusion, adjacent segment degeneration (ASD) can complicate an uneventful ACF with approximately a 25% risk of occurrence in the first ten postoperative years [10, 11]. Muscle-sparing tubular approaches for PCF have gained popularity, as

Electronic Supplementary Material The online version of this chapter https://doi.org/10.1007/978-3-319-71943-6_17. contains supplementary material, which is available to authorized users.

G.M. Ghobrial • A.D. Levi (✉)
Department of Neurological Surgery and The Miami Project to Cure Paralysis, Lois Pope LIFE Center, University of Miami MILLER School of Medicine, Miami, FL, USA
e-mail: georgeghobrial@gmail.com; Alevi@med.miami.edu

G. Tender (ed.), *Minimally Invasive Spine Surgery Techniques*,
https://doi.org/10.1007/978-3-319-71943-6_17

well as 'keyhole foraminotomy' approaches that allow for less-invasive corridor with microscopic or endoscopic assistance or in conjunction with a muscle-splitting tubular retractor.

Indications

Posterolateral soft disc herniation with concordant unilateral radicular symptoms.

Contraindications

Primarily axial neck pain symptoms, cervical subluxation, cervical kyphosis (<10°), severe spondylosis, and recurrent disc herniation, adjacent level disease with prior fusion at or above the level of index disease are all relative contraindications that should be weighed against a posterior foraminotomy approach. The presence of a calcified disc fragment or central disc herniation are contraindicated to the PCF technique.

Surgical Technique

The conventional open technique for the PCF has not changed over the previous 50 years [12]. However, modifications to accommodate 'muscle-sparing' technologies such as muscle-splitting tubular retractors, endoscopes, and operating microscope use, have decreased the morbidity of surgery [8, 13, 14]. After endotracheal intubation, total intravenous anesthesia is utilized to facilitate intraoperative neurophysiologic monitoring with continuous electromyography. Bite blocks are placed to avoid injury to the tongue if motor evoked potentials are utilized. The eyes are carefully taped shut to avoid corneal irritation from caustic skin prep or other debris. A Mayfield skull clamp is placed, and the patient is carefully turned prone with the head in the neutral position. The patient is secured to the radiolucent frame. Moderate traction is placed on the shoulders to aid in lateral fluoroscopic visualization of the disc level of interest and confirmation of ideal cervical alignment. Flexion of the head and neck can facilitate subsequent dissection and decrease the bony overhang between the lamina and facet of operative interest. Prior to draping, the skin incision is confirmed by fluoroscopy. The skin is disinfected with ethyl alcohol and then further with ChloraPrep® (2% chlorhexidine gluconate and 70% isopropyl alcohol; CareFusion, Inc., Leawood, KS) (Fig. 17.1).

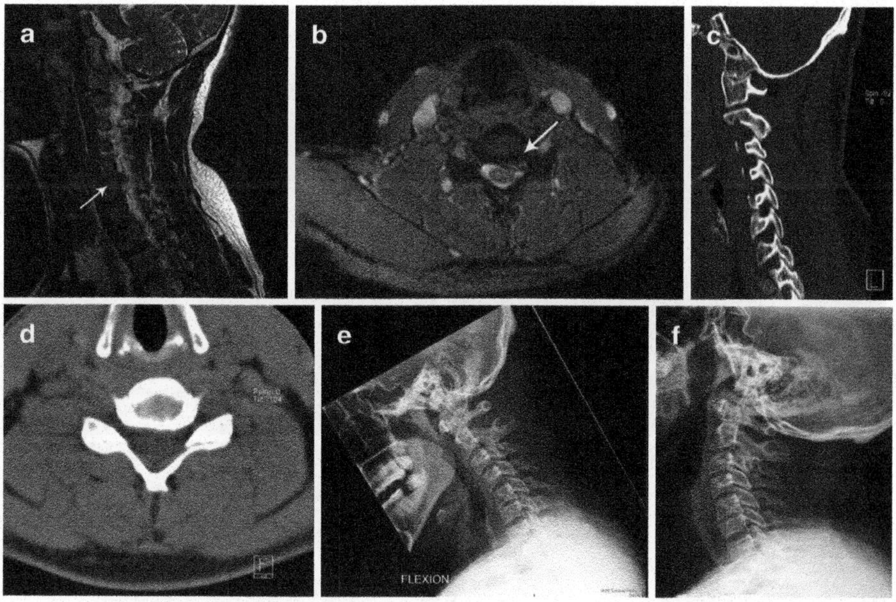

Fig. 17.1 Preoperative imaging findings in a 33 year-old female with left C6 radicular pain and a concordant C5/C6 posterolateral soft disc herniation on T2 MRI sagittal (arrow, **a**) and axial views (arrow, **b**) sequences. A CT was performed, ruling out the presence of a calcified disc (sagittal (**c**) and axial (**d**) which is a relative contraindication for a posterior cervical foraminotomy. The absence of subluxation on flexion (**e**) and extension (**f**) radiographs demonstrate no overt instability

Tubular-Approach

Tubular-access is performed at the surgeon's discretion and comfort level. The subsequent step-by-step approach using the Minimal Exposure Tubular Retractor System (METRx™, Medtronic, Minneapolis, MN) does not deviate greatly from the number of muscle-splitting retractors arriving on the market. The appropriate level of interest is localized first by lateral fluoroscopy to confirm the level and length of the skin incision, followed by anteroposterior (AP) fluoroscopy which is used to confirm that neck rotation is absent (Fig. 17.2a). Having an x-ray technician skilled in fluoroscopy of the spine is vital for limiting patient radiation to the head and radiosensitive soft tissues of the neck. Also, a true perpendicular view is needed to confirm a trajectory over the lateral mass and not the spinal canal. After marking the level of interest, the smallest inner tube in pressed on to the skin targeting the facet-lamina junction at the appropriate level and an imaginary line is drawn to help mark the skin. We avoid using the Steinman pin as an initial dilator to avoid inadvertent interlaminar entry (Fig. 17.2b). The starting point varies by the depth of soft tissue in the

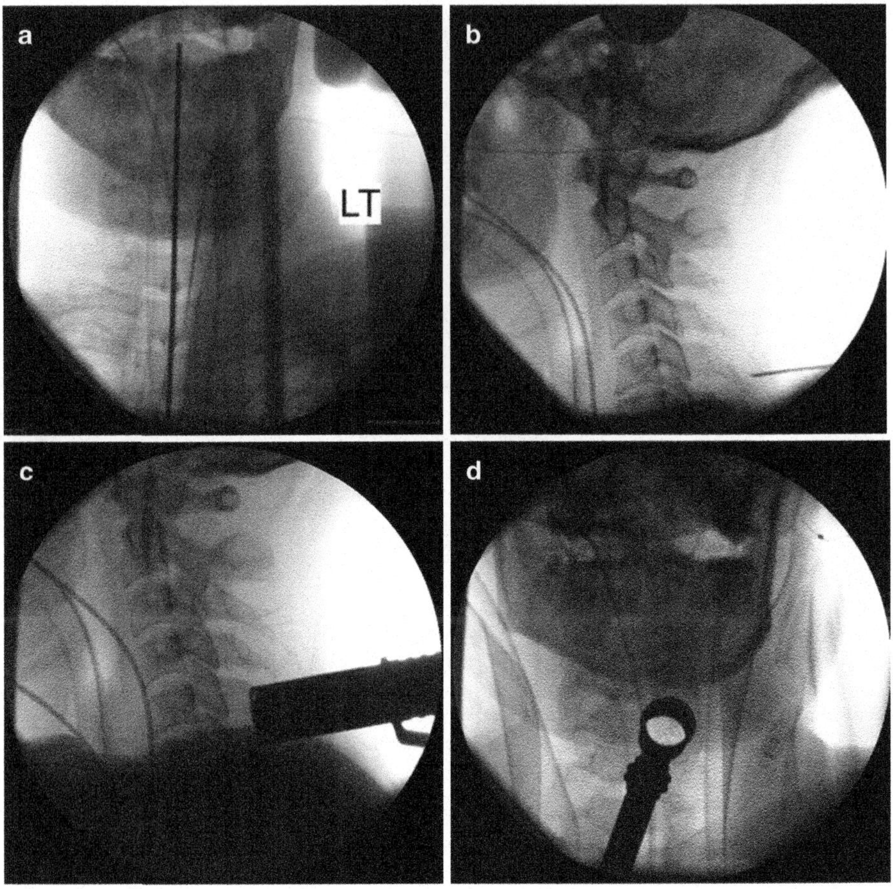

Fig. 17.2 Intraoperative Imaging Series. (**a**) Intraoperative fluoroscopy, anteroposterior (AP) view. The midline is marked with a K-wire, note the appropriate midline orientation spinous processes, without head or neck rotation. (**b**) Intraoperative fluoroscopy, lateral view. After a true lateral view is obtained, a 20-gauge needle is placed at a lateral entry point over the facet of interest (left C5–C6 facet) superficially over the facets, taking care not to enter into the canal. (**c**) Lateral fluoroscopic view confirming placement of the appropriate tube and removal of the dilators. The tube should be perpendicular to the entry point. (**d**) An AP fluoroscopic view is obtained demonstrating placement of the dilator over the C5–C6 facet. This is useful in confirming the appropriate orientation of the working channel with respect to midline

patient but is usually caudal to the target. It is extremely important to draw the line perpendicular to the ceiling so that the microscope is not tilted during the surgery. After subcutaneous injection of local anesthetic with epinephrine, a vertical skin incision is made to the desired length of the final tube (e.g. 16 mm for a 16 mm tube). The dorsal fascia may be incised as well. The smallest inner tube is now passed to the level of the fascia and the trajectory confirmed. Passing below the fascia increases risk of inadvertent injury to dura, nerve roots, or the spinal cord, and the operator can proceed at their level of comfort with regards to depth. The first dilator is carefully docked on the bony lamina/facet junction. Subsequent dilators are advanced to reach the desired final tube diameter (tubular length ranges from 3 to 9 cm with a diameter up to 18 mm) (Fig. 17.2c). An assistant now attaches the flexible arm to the bed rail distal to the cervical spine, opposite of the symptomatic side and the bed rail clamp is tightened by a nonsterile operating room assistant. The flexible arm is secured and the inner dilators may be removed. An AP x-ray can be obtained with the C-arm to confirm that the optimal lateromedial trajectory is maintained (Fig. 17.2d). This is performed prior to C-arm removal to help avoid inadvertent docking on bone too medial or lateral. Complete removal of soft tissue is essential to allow for the full use of the working corridor and can facilitate safe nerve root exposure.

Conventional-Approach

Patient anesthesia, positioning, and draping are done in the aforementioned technique. After localization with lateral fluoroscopy, a midline incision followed by unilateral subperiosteal dissection is performed. Exposure can be midline in smaller patients, aided by an avascular midline plane (ligamentum nuchae), which can decrease muscle bleeding and postoperative pain. In larger patients, a paramedian incision is desirable, as lateral foraminotomy access requires elongation of the midline incision, increasing posterior midline dissection and pain. Lateral radiography is obtained to confirm the appropriate spinal level. The lateral inferior edge of the rostral lamina and less than 50% of the medial facet are then exposed and removed with either a 3 mm diamond burr or a 1.8 mm fluted matchstick burr (Synthes Inc., West Chester, PA) with microscope-assistance [15]. A 1 mm Kerrison punch is used to resect the remaining cortical lamina, followed by the ligamentum. The axilla of the nerve root must be visualized and then exposed through careful bipolar cautery of epidural veins taking extreme caution to avoid heat transfer to the nerve root or thecal sac medially. Pediculotomy of the superomedial edge of the caudal pedicle has been described for further exposure, but is not routine [15]. Confirmation of adequate forminal decompression is performed by a right angle probe. After annular exposure, annolotomy can be performed with a No. 15 blade, followed by removal of compressive disc fragments in a piecemeal fashion. Postoperative imagine is not routinely performed, but can be obtain in the event of recurrent radicular symptoms with MRI, or in the case of new and persistent mechanical neck pain (Fig. 17.3).

Pearls and Pitfalls

1. *Wrong-level surgery*: This can result from a number of factors. Obesity and body habitus can result in poor fluoroscopic visualization due to obstruction of the lower cervical spine from the upper body and poor penetration of x-ray. Maximizing the distance of the head frame from the bed attachment allows for improved visualization of the lower cervical spine. A skilled x-ray technician can improve the contrast of the image by increasing x-ray penetration, eliminating artifact from scatter and

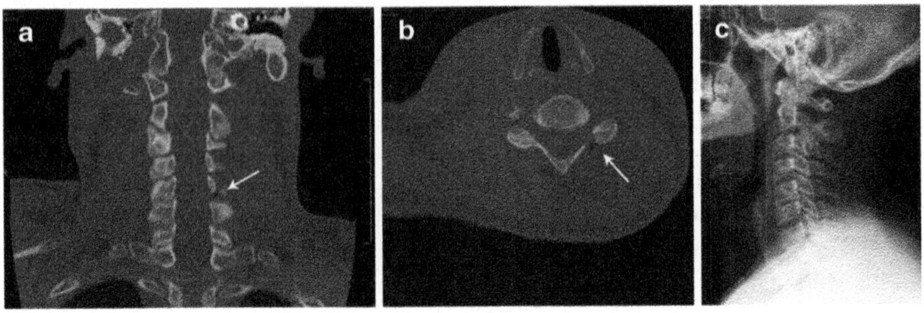

Fig. 17.3 Postoperative imaging in a 33 year-old female after left C5/C6 cervical foraminotomy. Work-up was performed by emergency department staff to exclude fracture from motor vehicle collision 2 days after surgery. Postoperative computed tomography of the cervical spine, coronal (**a**) and axial (**b**) views are presented. Postoperative air and resection of the lamina and medial facet is noted (arrows) Upright lateral radiograph (**c**) demonstrates maintenance of neutral alignment

parallax. Excessive spondylosis and facet or laminar overhang from a hyperkyphotic patient may require repeat confirmation of the appropriate level of interest. As previously mentioned, a fascial incision can help facilitate advancement of the K-Wires and dilator tubes to dock over the facet. It is a priority to understand the depth of these dilators at all times during advancement.

2. *Under-exposure*: The tendency with tubular or microscopic-assisted approaches is to perform a cone-shaped exposure, which can decrease visualization and increase operative duration. Removal of all soft tissue in the working channel with the underlying bone and ligamentum can allow for an expedient and safe discectomy and foraminotomy.
3. *Destabilization*: It is important to understand the bony landmarks of the patient prior to laminotomy and facetectomy. In the case of significant spondylosis, an AP radiograph can be confirmatory of proper tube positioning to limit extent of bony resection. Since the weight-bearing axis of the cervical spine is posterior to the vertebral bodies of C3–C6, the posterior tension is thought to maintain cervical lordosis. Therefore, aside from risk of subluxation by overly aggressive facetectomy, postlaminectomy kyphosis is a theoretical concern from foraminotomy. Ideally, the lamina should be identified first and the resection should proceed laterally to limit the extent of facetectomy and avoid destabilization [8]. Jagannathan et al. found a 4.9% rate of postoperative instability (8 patients) and only 1 patient was symptomatic and required fusion [8].

Complications

1. *Loss of Cervical Sagittal Alignment*: Retrospective data with 5-year radiographic follow-up has identified patients at risk for progression of cervical deformity after PCF. These include patients over 60 years of age, and less than 10° of preoperative cervical kyphosis. Treatment of deformity progression after

PCF or iatrogenic instability on flexion-extension films (i.e. subluxation) is commonly performed with either lateral mass fixation or ACF. One theoretical benefit of the tubular approach is that the minimal disruption of posterior musculature may preserve the tension band maintaining a neutral or lordotic cervical alignment. However, an anterior approach should be considered in a patient with cervical kyphosis, or cervical sagittal positive malalignment (C2–C7 plumb lines greater than 4 cm), as this should indicate a risk for worsening deformity.
2. *Nerve Root Injury*: Nerve root injury can occur in up to 10% of early open microscope-assisted PCF series [16]. Some authors advocate for a larger laminotomy and medial facetectomy in order to maximize visualization of the nerve root.

Selected Literature Review

Studies Comparing Posterior Cervical Foraminotomy to Anterior Cervical Discectomy and Fusion

1. Onimus et al. compared 14 patients with PCF to 14 patients after ACF with iliac crest bone graft (ICBG), finding no significant difference in patient reported outcomes (93% vs. 79% with good or excellent outcomes in the PCF and ACF groups, respectively) [17].
2. Herkowitz et al. compared ACF (n = 28) to posterior foraminotomy (n = 16) for soft disc herniation. 33 posterolateral disc herniations (ACF = 17, PCF = 16) and 11 central disc herniations (ACF = 11) were identified. Excellent or good pain relief and weakness was noted in 94% (16 of 17) in the ACF group and 75% (12 of 16) in the PCF group at 4 year follow-up. The authors conclude that ACF provides better long-term improvement [18].
3. Ruetten et al. randomized 175 patients to full endoscopic posterior foraminotomy or ACF with a polyetheretherketone (PEEK) cage (without plating) for lateral disc pathology in tandem with unrelenting radicular symptoms or neurologic deficit. No difference in clinical outcome at 2 years or complication rates were observed [13].

Selected Non-Comparative Posterior Cervical Foraminotomy Series

1. Henderson et al. reviewed 736 patients over a 20 year period and a mean follow-up of 2.8 years in patients that were treated with a PCF for a posterolateral soft disc herniation and cervical radiculopathy. All surgeries were done in the sitting position, 3% (n = 24) experienced recurrent radiculopathy and had a second operation. 92% of patients reported good or excellent postoperative symptomatic relief.

2. Jagannathan et al. reviewed 162 PCF cases with a 5 year follow-up finding a significant improvement in postoperative NDI in 93% of patients and resolution of radiculopathy in 95%. At a mean follow-up of 77 months, no significant changes in focal or segmental kyphosis, or disk height were observed with time. Loss of lordosis (greater than 10°) was seen in 30 patients (20%), but no significant trend towards cervical kyphosis was observed [8].
3. Skovrlj et al. followed 97 patients for a mean 32 months treated with minimally-invasive PCF using tubular dilators as described above. Significant improvements in the neck disability index and visual analog scale (neck and arm components) were observed [14].

Conclusions

The posterior cervical foraminotomy is a comparable surgical treatment for the relief of radiculopathy attributed to posterolateral soft disc herniation. Limited comparative prospective evidence is available comparing anterior cervical discectomy and fusion to posterior cervical foraminotomy.

References

1. Spurling RG, Segerberg LH. Lateral intervertebral disk lesions in the lower cervical region. J Am Med Assoc. 1953;151:354–9.
2. Raaf JE. Surgical treatment of patients with cervical disk lesions. J Trauma. 1969;9:327–38.
3. Murphey F, Simmons JC, Brunson B. Chapter 2. Ruptured cervical discs, 1939 to 1972. Clin Neurosurg. 1973;20:9–17.
4. Murphey F, Simmons JC, Brunson B. Surgical treatment of laterally ruptured cervical disc. Review of 648 cases, 1939 to 1972. J Neurosurg. 1973;38:679–83.
5. Fager CA. Management of cervical disc lesions and spondylosis by posterior approaches. Clin Neurosurg. 1977;24:488–507.
6. Fager CA. Posterior surgical tactics for the neurological syndromes of cervical disc and spondylotic lesions. Clin Neurosurg. 1978;25:218–44.
7. Samartzis D, Shen FH, Lyon C, et al. Does rigid instrumentation increase the fusion rate in one-level anterior cervical discectomy and fusion? Spine J. 2004;4:636–43.
8. Jagannathan J, Sherman JH, Szabo T, et al. The posterior cervical foraminotomy in the treatment of cervical disc/osteophyte disease: a single-surgeon experience with a minimum of 5 years' clinical and radiographic follow-up. J Neurosurg Spine. 2009;10:347–56.
9. Nandyala SV, Marquez-Lara A, Fineberg SJ, et al. Comparison between cervical total disc replacement and anterior cervical discectomy and fusion of 1 to 2 levels from 2002 to 2009. Spine. 2014;39:53–7.
10. Virk SS, Niedermeier S, Yu E, et al. Adjacent segment disease. Orthopedics. 2014;37:547–55.
11. Hilibrand AS, Carlson GD, Palumbo MA, et al. Radiculopathy and myelopathy at segments adjacent to the site of a previous anterior cervical arthrodesis. J Bone Joint Surg. 1999;81:519–28.
12. Scoville WB, Whitcomb BB. Lateral rupture of cervical intervertebral disks. Postgrad Med. 1966;39:174–80.

13. Ruetten S, Komp M, Merk H, et al. Full-endoscopic cervical posterior foraminotomy for the operation of lateral disc herniations using 5.9-mm endoscopes: a prospective, randomized, controlled study. Spine (Phila Pa 1976). 2008;33:940–8.
14. Skovrlj B, Gologorsky Y, Haque R, et al. Complications, outcomes, and need for fusion after minimally invasive posterior cervical foraminotomy and microdiscectomy. Spine J. 2014;14:2405–11.
15. Webb KM, Kaptain G, Sheehan J, et al. Pediculotomy as an adjunct to posterior cervical hemilaminectomy, foraminotomy, and discectomy. Neurosurg Focus. 2002;12:E10.
16. Williams RW. Microcervical foraminotomy. A surgical alternative for intractable radicular pain. Spine. 1983;8:708–16.
17. Onimus M, Destrumelle N, Gangloff S. Surgical treatment of cervical disk displacement. Anterior or posterior approach?. Rev Chir Orthop Reparatrice Appar Mot. 1995;81:296–301.
18. Herkowitz HN, Kurz LT, Overholt DP. Surgical management of cervical soft disc herniation. A comparison between the anterior and posterior approach. Spine. 1990;15:1026–30.

Chapter 18
Minimally Invasive Posterior Cervical Decompression

Mena G. Kerolus, Joseph E. Molenda, Mazda K. Turel, and Richard G. Fessler

Introduction

Minimally invasive surgical (MIS) procedures for posterior cervical laminectomy, laminoforaminotomy and discectomy techniques were developed to reduce muscle dissection and soft tissue trauma. MIS posterior cervical laminoforaminotomy has been shown to reduce operative times, blood loss, postoperative pain and duration of hospital stays. In carefully selected patients with lateral foraminal disease, excellent surgical results can be expected. In this chapter, we will discuss the indications, contraindications, surgical technique and common surgical nuances involved in a posterior cervical decompression. A video illustration of an MIS posterior cervical laminoforaminotomy is also included.

Indications

Patients who are candidates for MIS posterior cervical laminoforaminotomy typically present with unilateral pain, weakness, and/or sensory changes that involve the affected sensory or motor nerve root distribution. The most common cause of cervical radiculopathy is foraminal stenosis due to disc herniation and degenerative changes, which results in decreased disc height and foraminal stenosis. A prerequisite for patient selection is the combination of clinical signs and symptoms of

Electronic Supplementary Material The online version of this chapter https://doi.org/10.1007/978-3-319-71943-6_18. contains supplementary material, which is available to authorized users.

M.G. Kerolus • J.E. Molenda • M.K. Turel • R.G. Fessler (✉)
Department of Neurosurgery, Rush University Medical Center, Chicago, IL, USA
e-mail: Joseph_E_Molenda@rush.edu; rfessler@rush.edu

G. Tender (ed.), *Minimally Invasive Spine Surgery Techniques*,
https://doi.org/10.1007/978-3-319-71943-6_18

cervical radiculopathy with supporting radiographic findings. Patients with lateral foraminal disease are the best candidates for MIS posterior laminoforaminotomy. Mutli-level foraminal stenosis can also be addressed with an MIS posterior laminoforaminotomy. Furthermore, patients who have already had an anterior cervical discectomy and fusion (ACDF) with persistent radiculopathy are candidates for an MIS posterior cervical laminoforaminotomy. Patients with contraindications to proceeding with an ACDF are able to undergo an MIS posterior cervical laminoforaminotomy.

Contraindications

MIS posterior cervical laminoforaminotomy is contraindicated in patients with cervical kyphosis or cervical instability. Alignment and/or stabilization should be corrected prior to an MIS posterior cervical laminoforaminotomy. Cervical myelopathy is not treated with an MIS posterior cervical laminoforaminotomy alone. Additionally, patients with primarily ventral cord disease should not undergo an MIS posterior cervical decompression. Finally, paracentral or medial foraminal disc herniations that require any cord retraction should not undergo an MIS posterior cervical laminoforaminotomy. It is important to carefully evaluate for other symptoms that may mimic cervical radiculopathy including brachial plexopathies, nerve sheath tumors, inflammatory disorders, rotator cuff syndromes, or infectious etiologies.

Surgical Technique (Video 18.1)

Patients undergo general anesthesia in the standard fashion. Somatosensory evoked potentials and myotomal EMG monitoring will be used during surgery. While the procedure is frequently performed in the prone position, we recommend the semi-sitting position as it reduces bleeding and allows for blood to flow out of the surgical field, keeping it clean. After induction with general anesthesia, a three-point Mayfield head clamp is secured to the patient's head. The operating room table is then flexed so that the patient is in a sitting position with the neck perpendicular to the floor and the head slightly flexed. The Mayfield is secured to the table in front of the patient. The patient's arms and legs are padded to prevent any compression radiculopathies. The table head rest is then removed to expose the dorsal neck. A pillow under the buttocks is used to elevate the neck above the edge of the table back. The fluoroscopy arm is placed below the patient, with the base of the fluoroscopy unit on the same side as the planned incision. The x-ray beam should be in line with the patient's neck. The anesthesia station should be to the left of the surgeon, with the scrub table and monitors to the right side of the surgeon. Fluoroscopy is then used to determine the appropriate level.

The incision for an MIS posterior cervical foraminotomy is about 1.8–2.0 cm in length and 1.5 cm from midline. The incision is cut sharply and hemostasis achieved. The fascia is identified, then cut sharply under direct vision through the entire length of the incision. Metzembaum scissors are used to dissect through the paraspinal muscles, followed by the insertion of either a small or medium dilator to spread through the paraspinal muscles. It is very important to avoid any forceful downward pressure during dilation of the cervical paraspinal musculature because the cervical interlaminar space is wide and the dilators can easily plunge into the spinal canal. It is for this reason that we also do not recommend using a Kirschner wire, because if you are too medial, the risk of injuring the dura and/or spinal cord increases substantially. The ideal tubular docking location is on the facet itself. After docking, the tube is directed medially to expose the lamina-facet junction. The tubular retractor should be perpendicular to the lamina.

After securing the tubular retractors, the soft tissue is dissected in a lateral to medial direction. It is important to carefully identify the medial facet and the lateral edge of the lamina to avoid inadvertent injury to the spinal nerve root or spinal cord. The soft tissue is removed using pituitary rongeurs and the ligament visualized in the inferior medial aspect of the tube. An angled curette is carefully used to create a plane between the ligament and the undersurface of the lamina. Either a 1.0 or 2.0 mm Kerrison rongeurs is then used to remove the lamina. A drill can also be used to remove the lamina and medial facet. It is important to not remove more than 50% of the facet as this can cause instability of the cervical spine. Epidural veins will likely be encountered on the lateral edge of the ligament and along the nerve root and should be cauterized with bipolar forceps. A Kerrison rongeur is used in the inferior lateral direction to expose the nerve root. A nerve hook is then used to palpate the neural foramen to ensure adequate decompression both ventrally and dorsally. In general, if the hook can palpate the lateral aspect of the pedicle, adequate decompression has been achieved. Any osteophyte complex or disk herniation is removed with a slight mobilization of the nerve root. Upon completion of drilling, the ligament is removed using an angled curette and Kerrison. At this point, the lateral edge of the dura and proximal nerve root are observed under direct vision.

In cases of MIS posterior cervical laminectomy, the tubular retractor is rotated medially 30–45°. The soft tissues are removed. The ligament is again separated from the undersurface of the bone using an angled curette. The bone is then removed using a Kerrison punch and drill. It is important to keep the ligament intact as this provides a barrier when drilling the contralateral lamina. After decompression on the side of the initial approach, the tubes are directed medially to visualize the undersurface of the contralateral lamina. After bony decompression, the ligament is again removed using an angled curetted. Upon completion of drilling, the ligament is removed using an angled curette and Kerrison. At this point, the central dura mater should be decompressed and observed under direct vision.

Hemostasis is achieved using bipolar cautery and thrombin-soaked Gelfoam. The tubular retractors are slowly removed in a “stop and cauterize” fashion every few centimeters to address any bleeding. The fascia is then closed with 2-0 vicryl and the skin closed with 3-0 absorbable suture. Skin glue is to be used to seal the incision.

Postoperatively, patients recover in the postoperative bay and after general monitoring, are able to go home on the same day of surgery. At this point, patients can mobilize immediately.

Pearls and Pitfalls

- Especially in short patients, it is important to place a pillow under their buttocks to elevate their neck above the edge of the table back. The head rest portion of the table is removed to expose the dorsal neck.
- Forceful downward pressure should not be used during tubular dilation of the cervical paraspinal musculature. The fascia should be cut under direct vision, using Metzembaum scissors.
- Dock the tubes directly on the facet and angle medially as the last maneuver to expose the lamina-facet junction.
- Removal of more than 50% of the facet can result in cervical instability.
- In the sitting position, it is important that the head be slightly flexed and neck perpendicular to the floor. If the head is not correctly positioned, the surgeon will have difficulty viewing the appropriate anatomy and it will be ergonomically difficulty to perform the surgery. Correct alignment of the tube is also essential to keep blood out of the surgeon's view.
- The length of the incision should match the exact length of the dilating tube to help secure the tube and prevent unnecessary movement.
- After bony decompression, a nerve hook should easily pass ventrally and dorsally to the nerve root. The lateral edge of the spinal cord and proximal nerve root should be identified to ensure an adequate decompression was made.

Complications

Very few complications arise during an MIS posterior cervical laminoforaminotomy. However, there is a learning curve when performing MIS; hence, complications may occur early in the process.

Cerebrospinal fluid (CSF) leaks occur more commonly as the surgeon initially learns the procedure. Primary closure of the dura is generally not needed. Glue can be used as a dural-sealant and a tight closure of the fascia should avoid either a CSF leak or pseudomeningocele formation. In large dural tears, primary dural closure can be attempted. Postoperatively, a lumbar drain can be used for a few days if there is concern for a dural defect, although in our experience a lumbar drain is not needed.

Another common complication involves inaccurate docking of the tubular retractors. Incorrect placement of the tubular dilators can lead to disorientation and inappropriate drilling, further increasing the risk of neurologic injury. The ideal location for docking is the facet, which can be confirmed using fluoroscopy and an angled curette. Additionally, the cervical interlaminar space is wide; aggressive dilation can result in serious spinal cord injury if the dilators slip into this space. Fluoroscopy should be used on multiple occasions during dilation.

It is also important to be aware of anesthetic and positioning complications, especially when using the sitting position. Although air embolism is a possibility in the sitting position, it has rarely been observed when using tubular dilation for cervical laminoforaminotomy. A precordial doppler or transesophageal echocardiogram probe can be placed prior to incision to identify a venous air embolism. An air embolism can be identified by an increased endotracheal CO2 or hemodynamic changes can help indicate an air embolism. Venous congestion can also occur if the neck is flexed too much intraoperatively.

Literature Review

Open posterior cervical lamina decompression has been shown to be an effective method for treatment of cervical radiculopathy with up to 96% of patients reporting significant relief of arm pain and 98% of patients reporting resolution of motor deficits [1, 2]. MIS techniques were developed to decrease soft tissue destruction, blood loss, postoperative pain and subsequently shorter hospitalization times, while improving patient outcomes. However, for cervical radiculopathy, the gold standard has often been considered an open anterior approach with an ACDF. Although an ACDF can be used to treat foraminal stenosis and disc herniation, not all patients can tolerate an anterior approach given the risk of laryngeal injury, manipulation of the great vessels, and increased risk of airway edema and dysphagia.

Multiple clinical reports have demonstrated that MIS posterior cervical laminoforaminotomy and discectomy improves single-level cervical radiculopathy [3]. One and two-year prospective follow-up studies with patients undergoing MIS posterior cervical decompression have shown statistically improved neck disability index (NDI) and visual analog scale (VAS) neck and arm pain scores along with decreased blood loss, operative times and length of stay [4]. In a five-year prospective series of 70 patients who underwent a MIS posterior cervical foraminotomy with or without discectomy, Skovrlj et al. reported that only five patients (5.3%) required an ACDF after a mean of 44.4 months, three of whom required surgery at adjacent levels. NDI and VAS neck and arm scores were significantly improved, with that improvement lasting at least 5 years postoperatively [5]. Holly et al. evaluated 21 consecutive patients with cervical radiculopathy who underwent 2-level MIS posterior cervical foraminotomy. They found that 90% of patients had complete resolution of preoperative symptoms at a mean follow-up time of 23 months with no complications, suggesting that this MIS posterior cervical foraminotomy be a potential alternative treatment option for 2-level ACDF in selected patients [6].

Fessler et al. and Kim and Kim compared open and MIS posterior cervical laminoforaminotomy and found improved clinical outcomes and decreased hospitalization times, blood loss, and narcotic use in patients that underwent the MIS posterior cervical laminoforaminotomy [7, 8]. A prior systemic review demonstrated that MIS posterior cervical laminoforaminotomy reduced blood loss by 120 ml, decreased operative time by 50.0 min, resulted in less inpatient analgesia and resulted in a shorter length of stay (2 days) when compared to an open procedure [9]. However, one recent meta-analysis of open vs. MIS cervical foraminotomy found no significant differences in clinical outcomes, although both techniques were shown to have over a 92% clinical success rate [10]. MIS microscopic vs. endoscopic tubular decompression has been shown to have comparable operative times and complication rates. Both techniques were found to be significantly better in regards to hospitalization times, operative blood loss and postoperative analgesic requirements when compared to open treatment options [11].

Posterior cervical foraminotomy has been shown to be an effective treatment for cervical radiculopathy. In fact, most MIS posterior cervical techniques have been shown to be either equivalent, if not superior to open techniques. In order to prove clinical significance, MIS posterior cervical decompression has been compared to an ACDF, which has been regarded as the gold standard for cervical radiculopathy. Multiple studies have demonstrated that for the treatment of cervical radiculopathy, an ACDF or posterior foraminotomy demonstrate no significant differences in either patient outcomes or pain-relief [12]. Not only are clinical outcomes similar in patients undergoing MIS posterior cervical foraminotomy for single-level cervical radiculopathy or ACDF, but the mean direct total cost has been shown to be significantly less, which is largely due to the cost of the surgical implants [13]. Further supporting this, a recent systemic review of the literature for treatment of cervical radiculopathy concluded that MIS posterior cervical foraminotomy was just as safe and effective as ACDF for cervical radiculopathy, with some evidence that there were lower medical costs and a decrease in incidence of adjacent segment disease [14]. In a prospective, randomized, controlled study with a 2-year follow-up of 175 patients, similar clinical outcomes and VAS scores were reported in patients undergoing a full-endoscopic posterior foraminotomy or ACDF, while preserving mobility by avoiding instrumentation [15]. In a blinded, randomized, controlled trial, Soliman reported on a series of 70 consecutive patients with up to 3 levels of discogenic radiculopathy, myelopathy, or myeloradiculopathy in patients either undergoing cervical microendoscopic discectomy or ACDF. He found decreased complication rates, decreased postoperative analgesia requirements and shorter hospital stays in the cervical microendoscopic discectomy group [16]. In the most recent meta-analysis comparing randomized clinical trials using different treatment options (ACDF, cervical disc replacement, and MIS posterior cervical foraminotomy) for symptomatic single-level, cervical radiculopathy, MIS posterior cervical foraminotomy had the lowest rate of adverse events; however, there was no difference in which technique was the most effective nor which provided the longest-lasting relief from symptoms [17].

There has been recent interest in establishing MIS posterior cervical decompression techniques as a treatment for cervical myelopathy, inasmuch as open posterior cervical techniques have been shown to have greater immediate postoperative complications when compared to ventral decompression with ACDF [18]. In a recent retrospective review of 10 patients, Dahdaleh et al. reported that MIS posterior cervical decompression may be an effective treatment option for patients with cervical spondylotic myelopathy, for those patients with preoperative cervical lordosis. They demonstrated a statistically significant improvement in their Nurick score with no intraoperative or postoperative complications [19]. This was followed by another retrospective review of 74 patients comparing MIS posterior cervical decompression to ACDF for degenerative cervical myelopathy. Abbas et al. found comparable clinical outcomes, including NDI, VAS neck and arm pain, and similar minimal clinically important differences, while avoiding the need for cervical instrumentation [20].

Conclusion

MIS posterior cervical laminoforaminotomy provides an excellent treatment option for cervical radiculopathy in carefully selected patients. Appropriate patient positioning, an understanding of the posterior cervical anatomy, and careful surgical technique aid in successful surgical outcomes. MIS posterior cervical techniques have been shown to decrease hospitalization times, reduce blood loss and lower narcotic requirements. MIS posterior cervical decompression is similar in clinical efficacy to ACDF for the treatment of cervical radiculopathy and there is also some evidence that there is a decrease in associated costs. There is a learning curve when performing MIS, but with experience, both complications and operative times will decrease.

References

1. Henderson CM, Hennessy RG, Shuey HM, Shackelford EG. Posterior-lateral foraminotomy as an exclusive operative technique for cervical radiculopathy: a review of 846 consecutively operated cases. Neurosurgery. 1983;13(5):504–12.
2. Woertgen C, Holzschuh M, Rothoerl RD, Haeusler E, Brawanski A. Prognostic factors of posterior cervical disc surgery: a prospective, consecutive study of 54 patients. Neurosurgery. 1997;40(4):724–8.
3. Lidar Z, Salame K. Minimally invasive posterior cervical discectomy for cervical radiculopathy: technique and clinical results. J Spinal Disord Tech. 2011;24(8):521–4.
4. Lawton CD, Smith ZA, Lam SK, Habib A, Wong RHM, Fessler RG. Clinical outcomes of microendoscopic foraminotomy and decompression in the cervical spine. World Neurosurg. 2014;81(2):422–7.
5. Skovrlj B, Gologorsky Y, Haque R, Fessler RG, Qureshi SA. Complications, outcomes, and need for fusion after minimally invasive posterior cervical foraminotomy and microdiscectomy. Spine J. 2014;14(10):2405–11.
6. Holly LT, Moftakhar P, Khoo LT, Wang JC, Shamie N. Minimally invasive 2-level posterior cervical foraminotomy: preliminary clinical results. J Spinal Disord Tech. 2007;20(1):20–4.

7. Kim K-T, Kim Y-B. Comparison between open procedure and tubular retractor assisted procedure for cervical radiculopathy: results of a randomized controlled study. J Korean Med Sci. 2009;24(4):649–53.
8. Fessler RG, Khoo LT. Minimally invasive cervical microendoscopic foraminotomy: an initial clinical experience. Neurosurgery. 2002;51(5 Suppl):S37–45.
9. Clark JG, Abdullah KG, Steinmetz MP, Benzel EC, Mroz TE. Minimally invasive versus open cervical foraminotomy: a systematic review. Global Spine J. 2011;1(1):9–14.
10. McAnany SJ, Kim JS, Overley SC, Baird EO, Anderson PA, Qureshi SA. A meta-analysis of cervical foraminotomy: open versus minimally-invasive techniques. Spine J. 2015;15(5):849–56.
11. Winder MJ, Thomas KC. Minimally invasive versus open approach for cervical laminoforaminotomy. Can J Neurol Sci. 2011;38(2):262–7.
12. Wirth FP, Dowd GC, Sanders HF, Wirth C. Cervical discectomy. A prospective analysis of three operative techniques. Surg Neurol. 2000;53(4):340–6.
13. Mansfield HE, Canar WJ, Gerard CS, O'Toole JE. Single-level anterior cervical discectomy and fusion versus minimally invasive posterior cervical foraminotomy for patients with cervical radiculopathy: a cost analysis. Neurosurg Focus. 2014;37(5):E9.
14. Liu W-J, Hu L, Chou P-H, Wang J-W, Kan W-S. Comparison of anterior cervical discectomy and fusion versus posterior cervical foraminotomy in the treatment of cervical radiculopathy: a systematic review. Orthop Surg. 2016;8(4):425–31.
15. Ruetten S, Komp M, Merk H, Godolias G. Full-endoscopic cervical posterior foraminotomy for the operation of lateral disc herniations using 5.9-mm endoscopes: a prospective, randomized, controlled study. Spine. 2008;33(9):940–8.
16. Soliman HM. Cervical microendoscopic discectomy and fusion: does it affect the postoperative course and the complication rate? A blinded randomized controlled trial. Spine. 2013; 38(24):2064–70.
17. Gutman G, Rosenzweig DH, Golan JD. The surgical treatment of cervical radiculopathy: meta-analysis of randomized controlled trials. Spine. 2017. doi: 10.1097/BRS.0000000000002324. [Epub ahead of print].
18. Shamji MF, Cook C, Pietrobon R, Tackett S, Brown C, Isaacs RE. Impact of surgical approach on complications and resource utilization of cervical spine fusion: a nationwide perspective to the surgical treatment of diffuse cervical spondylosis. Spine J. 2009;9(1):31–8.
19. Dahdaleh NS, Wong AP, Smith ZA, Wong RH, Lam SK, Fessler RG. Microendoscopic decompression for cervical spondylotic myelopathy. Neurosurg Focus. 2013;35(1):E8.
20. Abbas SF, Spurgas MP, Szewczyk BS, Yim B, Ata A, German JW. A comparison of minimally invasive posterior cervical decompression and open anterior cervical decompression and instrumented fusion in the surgical management of degenerative cervical myelopathy. Neurosurg Focus. 2016;40(6):E7.

Chapter 19
D-TRAX

Clifford Crutcher, Anthony Digiorgio, Remi Nader, and Gabriel Tender

Introduction

Minimally invasive approaches have been extensively used in the lumbar spine, but less so in the cervical spine. Open posterior cervical approaches are particularly morbid, since the paraspinous muscles have to be detached from the spinous processes and laminae all the way out to the lateral edge of the lateral facets. The D-TRAX procedure has emerged as a great minimally invasive option in patients who need a posterior cervical fusion without a laminectomy.

Besides the obvious advantages of minimally invasive approaches, the D-TRAX procedure also seems to provide very high fusion rates, since the bone only needs to grow over a few mm and the cage is under axial loading, favoring Wolff's law. Moreover, the cages distract the facet joints in a parallel fashion, and thus there is no loss of lordosis

Electronic Supplementary Material The online version of this chapter https://doi.org/10.1007/978-3-319-71943-6_19. contains supplementary material, which is available to authorized users.

C. Crutcher • A. Digiorgio
Department of Neurosurgery, Louisiana State University Health Sciences Center, New Orleans, LA, USA
e-mail: ccrutc@lsuhsc.edu; Adigi2@lsuhsc.edu

R. Nader
Texas Center for Neurosciences PLLC, Houston, TX, USA

American Board of Neurological Surgery, Chicago, IL, USA

Department of Neurosurgery, University of Texas Medical Branch, Galveston, TX, USA

William Carey University, Hattiesburg, MS, USA

Department of Neurosurgery, Tulane University, New Orleans, LA, USA

G. Tender (✉)
Louisiana State University, New Orleans, LA, USA

G. Tender (ed.), *Minimally Invasive Spine Surgery Techniques*,
https://doi.org/10.1007/978-3-319-71943-6_19

after this procedure. Finally, the biomechanical stability offered by the D-TRAX cages appear to be similar to that offered by the lateral mass screws/rods constructs.

Indications

The D-TRAX procedure is FDA approved for patients with C3 through C7 cervical radiculopathy who have failed at least 6 weeks of conservative therapy, including rest, oral pain medication, physical therapy, and epidural steroid injections. Patients who have failed conservative therapy, continue to have severe pain, increasing weakness, or progressive loss of strength should be considered for surgery. Typical findings on clinical examination include concordant radicular symptoms, decreased reflexes, decreased strength, and decreased sensation. Patients usually have a positive Spurling sign, preoperative neck disability index score greater than or equal to 30, and preoperative neck and arm pain score (visual analogue score) greater than or equal to 6. Imaging findings (plain films, CT, or MRI) include disc degeneration, disc herniation, and loss of disc height.

We have also used the D-TRAX procedure in patients with multilevel anterior cervical fusions (with increased risk of pseudarthrosis) or with pseudarthrosis after ACDF.

Contraindications

In general, the D-TRAX procedure is contraindicated in patients with central stenosis, who have to undergo a laminectomy along with the fusion. Patients with cervical myelopathy, symptomatic central canal stenosis, kyphosis, obesity, advanced diabetes, or cancer of the spine should not undergo this procedure. Trauma patients with evidence of posterior ligament disruption also should not undergo the DTRAX procedure. Other contraindications include rapid joint disease, bone absorption, osteopenia or osteoporosis, active infection and local inflammation.

The D-TRAX procedure can also not be performed in patients in whom the level of interest cannot be visualized on the lateral fluoroscopic images.

Surgical Technique

Patient Positioning

The patient is placed in prone position with the arms tucked to the side and adequate padding for all pressure points (Video 19.1). The face is rested on the usual foam pad and occasionally we use 2-in. silk tape to stabilize the head and keep the hair out of the way. The taping, in the shape of a "U" letter, is started at one of the head corners of the table, passed over the suboccipital area with the hair pulled up, away from the cervical area, and then reattached to the other head corner of the table. The head should be placed in slight flexion and in a position as close to rotation-neutral as possible. We do not use the Mayfield head points or the horseshoe head rest because the connecting bar is in the midline and would interfere with the AP fluoroscopic images.

The next step is the placement of the shoulder pusher. This step is extremely important, since the operation cannot be done unless the targeted level is visualized on the lateral fluoroscopic image. In general, the number of levels visualized on the lateral image using the shoulder pusher is similar or slightly better than the preoperative lateral X-ray. The shoulder pusher is typically placed at the acromioclavicular joint level on each side and locked in position with the shoulders brought down as far as possible. In most patients, this allows for visualization of the C6–7 facet joints on the lateral image. It is important to remember that this maneuver stretches the brachial plexus on both sides and should not be employed for more than 15–20 min at a time. If the operation takes longer than that, we recommend releasing the pressure on the shoulders for a few minutes, before resuming the position. Moreover, once the cages at the lowest visualized level are inserted, we release the pressure on the shoulders and close the wounds (or insert additional cages at the more cranial levels, if necessary) with no stretching of the brachial plexus.

C-Arm Placement

The two C-arms are placed in a similar position as for an odontoid screw procedure. In order for the C-arms and the surgeon to have enough room, anesthesia has to be at the foot of the table and be forewarned that they will need longer tubing for the case. The lateral C-arm is first brought in with its' base at the right side of the patient (for a right-handed surgeon). Maintaining the lateral view, this C-arm is then swiveled towards the feet of the patient, to make room for the AP C-arm.

The AP C-arm is brought in from the top, in line with the OR table. Once in position, different angle AP views can be obtained by rotating the "C" of the C-arm. The most useful is the one in line with the facet joint of interest ("en face"), but unfortunately this cannot be maintained all the time, since the long instruments used during the procedure do not fit with the C-arm in this position.

Implant Insertion

The midline skin incision is about 1 cm long and typically located around the C7 or T1 spinous process. After local hemostasis, the skin is undermined with a hemostat on both sides of the spinous process. The 10-blade is used to make 2 incisions in the posterior cervical fascia, slightly cranial to the skin incision, one on each side of the spinous process. Up to 3 levels can be treated through the same skin incision, due to the lordotic shape of the cervical spine.

The procedure is continued using the dedicated D-TRAX instruments, which are used in the following specific sequence: the access chisel, the decortication trephine, the guide tube, the decortication rasp, the fork mallet, the decortication burr, the cage inserter, and the bone graft tamp.

The access chisel is used to bluntly penetrate the paraspinous muscles, targeting the facet joint of interest on both the AP and lateral fluoroscopic images. We recommend using two hands at all times when maneuvering these instruments, since they are long and minimal hand motions can result in large motions of the tip of the instrument. Once the tip of the access chisel reaches the posterior aspect of the facet joint, gentle tapping allows it to penetrate the posterior facet capsule and enter the joint; this is confirmed both by lateral fluoroscopy and a tactile feel. Occasionally, in patients with severe facet hypertrophy, the facet may be difficult to access; in these patients, we recommend starting on the caudal facet and slowly moving the tip of the chisel cranially, without losing contact with the bone, until the joint is encountered and entered. Once in the facet joint, an AP fluoroscopic image is obtained to confirm that the access chisel is in the middle of the joint, and then the chisel is advanced until its' tip comes in contact with the cranial pedicle; this typically projects 2–3 mm posterior to the posterior vertebral wall on the lateral fluoroscopic images. Care must be exercised during chisel tapping not to break the pedicle (Fig. 19.1).

The decortication trephine is then inserted over the access chisel and used to decorticate the posterior aspects of the superior and inferior facets. The teeth of the trephine are designed to cut only when rotated counterclock-wise. Therefore, we insert the trephine rotating clock-wise, to protect the muscle, and once we reach the bone (i.e., the posterior aspect of the facets), we start rotating counterclock-wise. Just a few rotations are sufficient.

The decortication trephine is then removed and the guide tube is inserted over the access chisel. Since the two teeth of the guide tube entering the facet joint are slightly thicker than the access chisel, once the guide tube is docked in the facet, the access chisel can be easily withdrawn. The assistant should stabilize the guide tube at all times by holding gentle downward pressure and not allow it to come out of the facet joint or migrate medially or laterally.

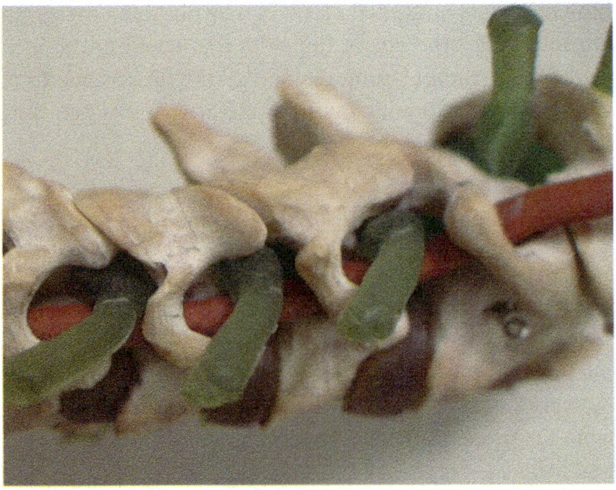

Fig. 19.1 Cervical spine model illustrating the local anatomy for D-TRAX insertion. The access chisel, advanced into the facet joint, will eventually hit the cranial pedicle

The decortication rasp is then inserted through the guide tube into the facet joint. The fork mallet is used to remove the decortication rasp and reinsert after turning 180° (this is done to decorticate both sides of the facet joint, since the rasp only has teeth on one side). The decortication rasp is reinserted a couple of times for each side of the facet. The decortication burr can also be used to increase the depth of decortication.

All the maneuvers described are performed under frequent lateral and AP fluoroscopic guidance, and using two hands to control the instruments and ensure the medial or lateral facet capsule is not violated.

The cage is then packed with graft material of choice and inserted into the joint using the cage inserter until the tip of the cage touches the cranial pedicle. Optionally, a bone screw can be inserted through the cage and into the superior facet, to maximize stability. The adequate cage position should be confirmed prior to insertion of the bone screw, since bone screw insertion is an irreversible step (i.e., once inserted, it cannot be removed using the D-TRAX instruments). The cage inserter is then detached from the cage and removed. Additional graft material is placed over the prepared bony surfaced of the lateral masses to promote fusion.

The opposite level, as well as any additional levels, is treated as indicated, through the same small skin incision. The wound is then copiously irrigated and closed in layers. There is no need for meticulous hemostasis of the muscle, since the muscle was dissected using blunt instruments. Moreover, no neural tissue is at risk of compression by a possible postoperative hematoma. We often inject Exparel into the paraspinous muscles for postoperative pain control.

Pearls and Pitfalls

This is a relatively safe technique with straightforward operative steps and little morbidity. If good AP and lateral fluoroscopic images can be obtained, the actual operation, skin to skin, should take about 15–20 min per level. As mentioned above in the surgical technique, controlling the long instruments with two hands and taking frequent fluoroscopic shots are useful tips to keep the instruments in the joint without violating the medial or lateral capsule. Violent tapping of the access chisel may lead to the theoretical risk of breakage of the cranial pedicle, although we have not seen or heard anybody having this complication so far.

Complications

Wrong Level Surgery

The only way this can happen is if, on the lateral fluoroscopic image, the facet joint on one side is lined up with the facet joint of the above or below level on the other side. Once the facet joint is penetrated with the access chisel, that facet HAS to be fused, even if it's the wrong level.

Medial Misplacement

In case of gross medial misplacement, the spinal cord can be injured, with resultant hemi or quadriparesis. However, if the medial capsule is just barely breached and the dura is not violated, it is unlikely that the patient will experience radiculopathy, since the corresponding nerve is typically located more caudal. If the patient is symptomatic, the cage can be removed using a tubular retractor to only expose that facet joint. The high-speed drill is used to remove enough bone from the facets to remove the cage, and then a single level lateral mass screw—rod construct is used to complete the fusion. The same technique can be applied using an open unilateral exposure with midline incision.

Lateral Misplacement

The danger of violating the lateral facet capsule is that the cage may become loose in the facet joint. If the violation of the lateral capsule is recognized intraoperatively, usually after careless manipulation of the access chisel, we attempt to place the cage slightly more medial than usually, and add the bone screw for stability.

Pedicle Fracture

Violent tapping of the access chisel may lead to the theoretical risk of breakage of the cranial pedicle, although we have not seen or heard anybody having this complication so far. The risk is increased by the fact that the vertebral artery lies on the other side of the pedicle and can thus be injured.

Cage Retropulsion

This complication may arise if the cage has not been inserted deep enough and the back of the cage is outside the facet joint. While we have not seen this complication in our series, it is likely that cage retropulsion remains asymptomatic, since there are no neural structures at risk in the region.

Pseudarthrosis

We have not seen this complication in our series either. If there is evidence of symptomatic pseudarthrosis, a standard open approach with lateral mass screws/rods can be used as a salvage procedure.

Literature Review

This is a relatively new technique [1] and therefore the relevant literature is scarce.

Initial biomechanical studies showed good stability after cage insertion [2–4].

Clinical studies confirmed good clinical results [5–9], although prospective studies and long-term results are not available.

Conclusion

The D-TRAX procedure offers an excellent alternative for posterior cervical fusion in selected patients.

References

1. McCormack BM, et al. Percutaneous posterior cervical fusion with the DTRAX facet system for single-level radiculopathy: results in 60 patients. J Neurosurg Spine. 2013;18:245–54. https://doi.org/10.3171/2012.12.spine12477.
2. Voronov LI, et al. Bilateral posterior cervical cages provide biomechanical stability: assessment of stand-alone and supplemental fixation for anterior cervical discectomy and fusion. Med Devices. 2016;9:223–30. https://doi.org/10.2147/mder.s109588.
3. Voronov LI, Siemionow KB, Havey RM, Carandang G, Patwardhan AG. Biomechanical evaluation of DTRAX((R)) posterior cervical cage stabilization with and without lateral mass fixation. Med Devices. 2016;9:285–90. https://doi.org/10.2147/mder.s111031.
4. Leasure JM, Buckley J. Biomechanical evaluation of an interfacet joint decompression and stabilization system. J Biomech Eng. 2014;136:071010. https://doi.org/10.1115/1.4026363.
5. Smith W, Gillespy M, Huffman J, Vong V, McCormack BM. Anterior cervical pseudarthrosis treated with bilateral posterior cervical cages. Oper Neurosurg. 2017. https://doi.org/10.1093/ons/opx103.
6. Skovrlj B, Qureshi SA. Minimally invasive cervical spine surgery. J Neurosurg Sci. 2017; 61:325–34. https://doi.org/10.23736/s0390-5616.16.03906-0.
7. Siemionow K, Monsef JB, Janusz P. Preliminary analysis of adjacent segment degeneration in patients treated with posterior cervical cages: 2-year follow-up. World Neurosurg. 2016;89(730):e731–7. https://doi.org/10.1016/j.wneu.2016.01.053.
8. Siemionow K, et al. Clinical and radiographic results of indirect decompression and posterior cervical fusion for single-level cervical radiculopathy using an expandable implant with 2-year follow-up. J Neurol Surg A Cent Eur Neurosurg. 2016;77:482–8. https://doi.org/10.1055/s-0036-1584210.
9. Siemionow K, Janusz P, Glowka P. Cervical cages placed bilaterally in the facet joints from a posterior approach significantly increase foraminal area. Eur Spine J. 2016;25:2279–85. https://doi.org/10.1007/s00586-016-4430-7.

Index

G. Tender (ed.), *Minimally Invasive Spine Surgery Techniques*,
https://doi.org/10.1007/978-3-319-71943-6

The manufacturer's authorised representative in the EU is Springer Nature Customer Service Centre GmbH, Europaplatz 3, 69115 Heidelberg, Germany. If you have any concerns regarding our products, please contact ProductSafety@springernature.com

Printed and bound by CPI Group (UK) Ltd, Croydon, CR0 4YY
30/09/2026
02225435-0001